THE
EVERYDAY
MEDICAL
HANDBOOK

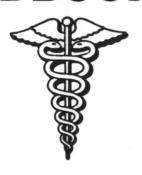

By George C. Thosteson, M.D.

In Collaboration with Jack Pickering

Fifth Printing

CONTENTS

Material in this book is reprinted from "To Your Good Health,"
published by Publishers-Hall Syndicate, Copyright © 1964, 1965, 1966, 1967, 1968.

EDITOR: FRANK BOWERS

Larry Eisinger, editor-in-chief; George Tilton, managing editor;
Silvio Lembo, art director; Harold E. Price, assoc. art director;
Elaine E. Sapoff, production editor

Printed in the United States of America by Fawcett Printing Corp., Rockville, Maryland

Introduction

ALTHOUGH THIS BOOK includes hundreds of subjects and is indexed according to topic, it is not intended to be an encyclopedia. That would require too many pages — and for a great many people would cost more than they could afford to spend. A whole book, or indeed quite a few books, could be written on any single chapter of this book. Just visit a medical library!

Rather, this book seeks to put at the reader's fingertips the answers to questions which arise in the lives of average families. The items, the questions and answers, have been compiled from the thousands that have appeared in my newspaper column over the last 15 years and more. Most, actually, are from the more recent years, and brought up to date where necessary.

I have tried not to clutter it up with answers to questions that in general everybody knows anyway, nor to include too much about extremely rare or specialized problems.

Rather, I have tried to include answers to questions which come up quite frequently in American life — but questions to which the average layman does *not* know the answer. Quite a few million letters have passed over my desk, sometimes at the rate of 750,000 or more in a single year. These letters have been my guide as to what to try to include in this book.

This is not a "textbook," and not a medical dictionary. It is simply a book designed to answer the health questions that a great many people are asking, in many instances questions which folks' own doctors do not have time to answer day after day.

It includes questions which come to me repeatedly with the comment, "I know you've written about this before — but at the time I didn't think I would need the information for myself, so I didn't save your column."

My suggestion, therefore, is that you read the whole book, a little at a time, so you will have a general idea of what it contains and where.

Then, when a specific problem comes up, refer to the index in the back of the book, for the page numbers.

I hope that readers will accept this book in the same way they have accepted the newspaper column — an estimated 20,000,000 a day accepting me in my role of doctor talking to patients and friends; not giving lectures, not talking in medical jargon which, while invaluable to a physician, is often gibberish to anyone else; just a doctor talking in plain language about problems that puzzle, baffle or frighten all of us.

Pregnancy & Women's Problems

THERE IS ONE point above all others that I hope to make in this chapter, so far as pregnancy is concerned. For safety, and for the sake of healthy babies, there is no substitute for starting medical care *just as soon as a woman knows or suspects she is pregnant.*

Americans and Canadians have properly-famed medical facilities, and high standards of health. Yet our infant mortality figures are too high, higher than in quite a few less prosperous countries of the world. Why? The big reason is the too-well-rooted idea that it is all right to wait for months, and make arrangements to see the doctor only a few weeks, sometimes a few days, before the baby is expected to be born.

Too many times, some problem of excessive weight, faulty diet, swelling of the ankles or sometimes a very dangerous condition such as, perhaps, liver, heart or kidney ailment, or even toxemia, has developed which should be treated early.

Postponing the first visit to the doctor is not an economy. Physicians generally set a "package price" for a pregnancy and delivery, whether care begins early or late in the pregnancy. Go early; it costs no more, and it guards health, yours and the baby's.

My daughter-in-law had bleeding when she was three months pregnant. Examination shows that the baby is dead but the doctor says she must wait (perhaps a day, a week, or even a month or two) and expel the baby by herself.

Why must the mother carry a dead baby that long? It seems cruel. Why can't they take it from her?

I agree that it seems cruel, but there are good reasons. It is impossible to predict exactly when Nature will take its course and expel the fetus, but it usually is safest to wait.

One reason is the danger of infection being introduced in taking the fetus surgically. (Even though the fetus is dead, there is no infection present in the uterus.)

A second reason is that the uterus is losing its tone, and increased danger of hemorrhage exists if surgery is attempted.

The mother, while waiting, should be watched carefully, however. Certain blood tests will keep track of changes in the clotting ability of her blood (its ability to form fibrin) and if too much change is noted in clotting power, special efforts are made, either by drugs or surgery, to hasten expulsion of the fetus.

The situation is complicated, and you must rely on your physician's judgment.

Can you give me some information about exercises for pregnant women? I am four months pregnant and concerned about staying fit.

Exercise is important in keeping fit, but there are other reasons besides. One is to help keep weight under control. Another is that it makes for easier deliveries.

You are (I take it) seeing your doctor, and I much prefer that you direct this question to him. There are variations in doctors' preferences. More important, there are individual differences in patients which at times may have a bearing on the amount of exercise. A woman who has had previous miscarriages must be more restrained in physical activity, for one instance.

In general, however, any reasonable exercise short of tiring yourself is excellent. Walking outdoors is easiest and perhaps best, all things considered, since it can be continued throughout the pregnancy.

In the earlier and middle months simple calisthenics (bending, leg-raising, arm motions) should be safely tolerated by a healthy woman. Even swimming is acceptable, or golf if you like it although I would limit it to nine holes. Or bowling so long as it isn't tiring.

As the pregnancy progresses, the more active exercise becomes cumbersome and an effort, which takes care of the matter automatically. But there is still walking.

A little over a year ago I had my first baby, by Caesarean section. I was told then that any future births would have to be by the same method. I am now 30. Since I want another child, would it be wiser to wait a few years, and would a Caesarean then be less dangerous?

Generally speaking, there is no safety in waiting. It is better to have your babies early in life (in the 20's preferably). If there is some special consideration in your case, your doctor will tell you so. (I believe the record, if you want to call it that, is 13 Caesarean births for one mother.)

Can a virgin become pregnant? I stopped my boy friend before we went all the way, but now my period is late and my friends tell me I could be pregnant. I've prayed and am scared and awfully nervous.

This question comes up often enough to make it obvious that the younger generation, supposedly so sophisticated, misses the point about "going all the way."

Pregnancy can occur whenever an ovum, or female egg cell, is present, and is penetrated by a male sperm cell. Although an emission contains millions of sperm cells, only one is needed for pregnancy.

"Going all the way" is a somewhat vague term, but the important question is whether just one sperm cell found its way into the vaginal tract and to the ovum. These cells are vigorous and can "swim" or be carried quite a distance through the vaginal area. Such pregnancies probably are rare but they are possible, and every girl should be told of this possibility.

I have been chided at times as being a square old fogey for insisting that chastity is not an out-of-date virtue. The foregoing letter is typical of many that I receive from girls who are anxious, frightened or remorseful when they learn or suspect that sexual "freedom" isn't as simple and safe as they had let themselves suppose.

The sexual drive exists to procreate the race. Any sexual experimentation or byplay that permits the sperm cell to reach an ovum permits Nature to take its course and cause pregnancy. Yes, a "virgin" can become pregnant.

My mother says a woman can get pregnant while menstruating, and that the children will be crippled or deformed. I told her this is impossible but she disagrees.

Pregnancy then is not possible.

Doctors have run every imaginable test on my husband and me to learn what is preventing us from becoming parents. We are both fertile individuals and have been married five years. The doctors suggest that I undergo an exploratory operation. What can they find out from this? I am 24 years old.

I'm glad that your husband has been tested, too. Failure to conceive is not always the woman's fault; one-third to one-half the cases of infertility involve the man.

"Infertility" is usually regarded as meaning that pregnancy does not occur after a year or two of marriage. Yet the fact remains that considerable more time may pass — and several years later pregnancy DOES sometimes occur.

After prior illnesses have been studied, glandular deficiencies corrected, physical defects repaired, occasionally a marriage still remains childless and without any reason. This proves, of course, that we don't know all the answers.

At times an incompatibility of blood type (I don't mean the Rh factor) is reflected in the sperm; this can prevent conception. It has been shown that sensitivity may occur in the wife to the male sperm.

Too much effort may exhaust the male potential, and a rest can prove to be the best solution.

Psychological factors are important; anxiety rises over "infertility" as the months pass. The greater the worry, the greater the difficulty in achieving pregnancy, and it is not too unusual for couples, giving up hope, to adopt a baby — and then have children of their own once their nerves have relaxed.

What can surgery do? A small fibroid may be found. Endometriosis, which can prevent pregnancy, can be detected more accurately by surgical exploration. It is a rather common cause of infertility.

Unsuspected developmental defects may be found and possibly corrected. Likewise a procedure called a "wedge resection" may be performed on the ovaries, and this sometimes increases fertility.

But I also recommend, once again, a prescription that perhaps is not used often enough — a relaxing vacation. This often works.

Must a new diaphragm be used after birth?

After childbirth, it is often necessary to have a different diaphragm fitted. Don't trust the old one unless your doctor has found it to fit properly.

My sister says a woman's safe days are 14 days before her period. I say it's 14 days afterwards. What do you say?

By "safe days," you mean the time when pregnancy cannot occur.

It so happens that the fertile and infertile times in the cycle are not nearly as exact as some people think — or some wish. For pregnancy the ovum or egg must first emerge from the ovary. Then it must be fertilized within a reasonably short time by the male sperm.

For women with very regular cycles, the time of ovulation tends to follow a more or less steady pattern. For irregular cycles, ovulation isn't so easy to predict. But regardless of the duration of the cycle, it is thought that ovulation, and hence the fertile period, generally occurs 14 days or so before the beginning of the next menstrual period.

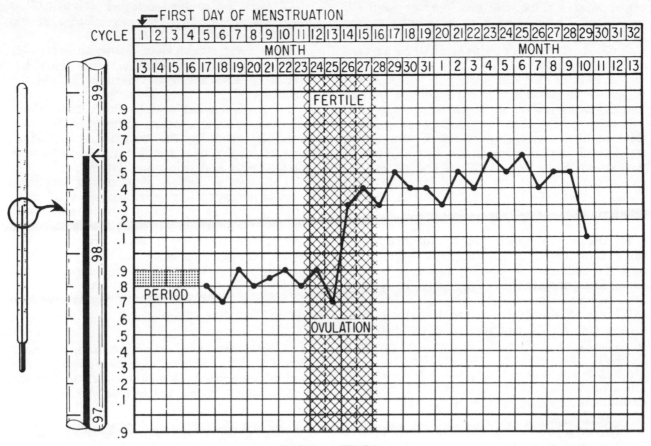

FIRST DAY OF MENSTRUATION

CYCLE	1	2	3	4	5	6	7	8	9	10	11	12	13	14	15	16	17	18	19	20	21	22	23	24	25	26	27	28	29	30	31	32
MONTH																				MONTH												
	13	14	15	16	17	18	19	20	21	22	23	24	25	26	27	28	29	30	31	1	2	3	4	5	6	7	8	9	10	11	12	13

RHYTHM METHOD

Thus in a perfectly regular 28-day cycle, ovulation would occur around the 14th day after the beginning of the preceding period, or 14 days before the beginning of the next one.

The latter probably applies for the 35-or 45-day cycles — 14 days before the NEXT one. But knowing when the next one will start isn't so easy.

The life of the ovum or egg is probably about 48 hours; life of the male sperm cell may be somewhat longer. Therefore the time during which pregnancy may occur can extend over three or four days.

How does one dry up the breasts after nursing a baby? I have nursed mine for six months, and plan to discontinue in about four more.

The flow of milk depends on your good health plus continued, regular nursing. When the baby is to be weaned, the frequency of suckling is reduced gradually and eventually stopped. You can omit one breast feeding each day, or every other day, substituting, of course, a bottle feeding. The flow of milk then decreases rapidly and automatically.

The breasts may become swollen and sore at this time, but the discomfort subsides in a few days and they return to normal.

A firm (not necessarily tight) support, as a brassiere, may ease the discomfort during these few days, but no other precautions are necessary.

Ever since the birth of my baby, I have begun losing hair at such a rate that I will soon be almost bald unless I can do something to stop it. My doctor tells me not to worry about it, but how can I help worrying? I am only 23.

This occurs occasionally after childbirth, and the assumption is that some change in hormone balance is responsible, although the exact process remains a mystery.

It comes as a shock, I admit — but the fact remains that this is usually a temporary thing. Although it may take several months, the hair grows in again.

There sometimes is hair loss after an operation requiring anesthesia, but that also corrects itself.

It is entirely different from hair loss from skin diseases, or from "pattern baldness," which is essentially a hereditary matter about which we can do nothing.

I am two months pregnant. I have already gained 15 pounds. Ordinarily I do not have any tendency to gain excess weight.

My doctor says: "Fine. You're eating for two." But I don't agree; it's too much. With seven months to go, can you imagine what I'll look like? There is nothing physically wrong with me, only a tremendous appetite. I am sure I can control this, but will the baby be harmed if I stay on a low calorie diet?

A gain of 18 to 20 pounds in pregnancy is regarded as normal; your 15 pounds in two months is, as you think, too much.

Odd quirks can accompany pregnancy. Occasionally overweight is the result of too much fluid accumulating in the womb, but most women would be better off not to look for excuses, but to do as you do and face the plain facts. Sometimes the appetite starts to run away — the only answer is call a halt to it.

You are "eating for two," but when you start gaining too much weight, you are eating more than the two of you need — one adult and one very tiny developing baby.

The essential needs of the baby are protein, vitamins, calcium and iron. Lean meat and eggs take care of the first, the protein. A quart of milk a day amply provides calcium plus some protein and a supply of fat — if weight is a problem, skim milk can be substituted. It is quite common to give pregnant women vitamins and iron and sometimes calcium (if they won't drink milk) to stay on the safe side.

In early pregnancy how long is it safe to wear a regular girdle or garter belt?

First, so far as the baby is concerned, you don't have to worry about him or her. He is well protected inside, and any exterior pressure would become annoying to you long before it could possibly harm the baby.

Second, the danger from tight girdles, garters or other garments which restrict surface circulation, involves formation of varicose veins, since in general veins are near the surface of the body (arteries are deeper).

The majority of women don't get varicose veins from pregnancy, no matter what they wear. A minority — meaning those who have fragile veins, or for some other reason show signs of developing varicose veins at childbearing age — should be careful.

Does a blue vein mean it is varicose? Not necessarily. How do you know whether a blue vein is or isn't varicose? The only reliable way is to ask your doctor.

Third, don't interpret anything I have said as meaning that girdles or garter belts are harmful, if you use ordinary good judgment. When you begin to find that your regular girdle is getting too snug for comfort, that's the time to change to a special one, or maternity girdle, which can be adjusted as needed. It will, if you'll accept the terminology, give support fore and aft, and will be most helpful in taking strain off the small of your back. After all, when you are carrying a baby, it changes your balance, and that puts added strain on certain muscles, especially those in the back.

I have an underdeveloped uterus. What does this mean? Is there any chance of my ever having children? I love them.

The term means that the organ is smaller than average for an adult woman. "Infantile uterus" is also sometimes used as an apt description.

There's a great deal we don't know about why some people develop differently, but this particular condition has been found in certain constitutional types: for instance, women with small breasts and thin musculature.

As to your chances of becoming pregnant, I am through with predictions. If your menstrual pattern is reasonably normal and ovulation occurs, pregnancy is quite possible. On the other hand, if there is some glandular deficiency, fertility may be impaired.

Many a woman with an undersized uterus has been told that she "couldn't have children," but when a healthy bundle of joy arrives, the doctors' face has turned red.

I maintain there is no pregnancy longer than 280 days, only a miscalculation on the part of the mother. Is a 10½-month pregnancy a possibility? Please settle this argument for me.

I hope you aren't in a hair-pulling match with anyone over this. An error of a couple of weeks in estimating duration of a pregnancy is commonplace. Any doctor will tell you that some women can be a bit hazy about the exact date of the last period. Besides that, the exact time of ovulation can vary.

In any event, 280 days is the AVERAGE length of pregnancy. Texts on obstetrics refer to some much longer than that, the longest I find mentioned being 331 days.

Is breast-feeding detrimental to a woman's figure?

No. Sagging seems to be due to loss or increase of weight rather than breast-feeding.

I have heard that the milk supply diminishes to nothing if birth control pills are taken. Is this true? Since I have had no period since my baby was born, can I just start taking the pills any time?

Yes, it is true. If you want to maintain a full milk supply, you must forego the pills. Your periods eventually will resume; then you will have a guide as to the proper time to use birth control pills.

What about the marking or "pregnancy veil" which bothers a lot of women who take "the pill" for contraception?

Is there any lotion on the market to fade this darkening for us vain people?

This darkening of the skin is called chloasma (clo-AZ-muh) and was dubbed "the mask of pregnancy" long before the pill was invented.

It is a darkening which occurs, in some women, when they are pregnant and fades out afterward.

Now it is being noticed in some women who use the pill — and since the pill causes the endocrine system to take on the characteristics that occur in pregnancy, this "false pregnancy" evidently misleads the skin tissues, and they react as they would in a real pregnancy. As I said, not all women are subject to this; just some.

As the discoloration fades at termination of a pregnancy, it also may fade when the pill is discontinued — although apparently it may take quite a bit of time.

Anyway, sometimes the marks are quite persistant, and naturally cause more concern if they happen to appear on the face.

If they don't fade, I understand that dermatologists have an ointment, containing monobenzone, which can get rid of the marks. This ointment can be irritating to normal skin, hence must be prescribed by and used under the direction of someone who understands proper use of it — meaning a skin specialist.

I am four months pregnant and about every six weeks I have a period, or threat of miscarriage.

My doctor recommends bed rest when this bleeding occurs. He tells me to stay off my feet and possibly I may be able to carry the child the full nine months. He also mentioned that the afterbirth seems to be first.

What effect can this periodic bleeding do to my unborn baby, and what if the afterbirth is first?

I have heard so many tales that I am quite upset — that the baby may not live, or if it does it will be a moron, or very small and sickly. What are the chances of my having a normal child?

From the description, there evidently is a threat of miscarriage, and the usual treatment is just what your doctor has advised — bed rest.

However if the baby is born successfully, neither condition — that is, early or late bleeding — affects the formation or intelligence of the child. Ignore the tales you hear. Some people delight in telling such distressing fabrications. Just pay attention to your doctor's counsel.

As to the afterbirth question, I assume this to mean that the placenta (which later becomes the afterbirth) is located at or near the opening of the womb, instead of higher up.

This is called placenta previa, that is, the placenta is so located to be in advance, instead of behind, the baby at the time of birth. It is an additional problem to be contended with at the time of delivery, but your doctor has detected it already, and the old maxim holds true here: Forewarned is forearmed.

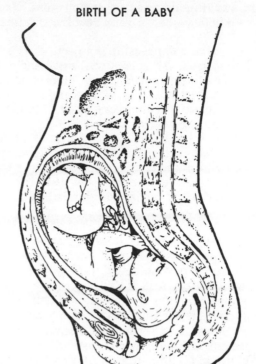

BIRTH OF A BABY

At the beginning of birth and height of uterine contraction, uterus exerts pressure on the amnion, which forces birth canal to open, permits head to drop down.

Will a tooth X-ray (two pictures) when I was about six days pregnant affect my baby?

Radiation can be harmful. This we must accept. The amount of radiation is vastly important. A little is of no consequence. Too much can be harmful.

So what about dental X-rays? The exposure is brief; the rays are aimed at the teeth, not at the fetus — the baby which is being formed.

Total irradiation of the body is one thing. Irradiation of a limited area is quite another. Use of X-rays so that they penetrate the womb in pregnancy is to be done only with great caution and under conditions of urgent need. (It also makes a difference whether the X-ray is used when the baby's body is in the formative stage, or has come close to being ready for birth.)

Thus while X-rays of the abdomen could carry a risk early in pregnancy, X-rays of a broken leg — or X-rays of teeth — do not involve any such risk to the baby.

I had a nervous breakdown after the birth of my first child, and the doctors called it postpartum depression. A book on the subject suggests thyroid for it, sometimes accompanied by shock treatments. Would you discuss?

Thyroid is frequently helpful in postpartum depression. Shock therapy is not usually needed and is not as effective in this type of depression as in others.

Such depression, or emotional illness, occurs in varying degrees of seriousness. From 4,000 to 5,000 women a year require treatment for it.

Post-partum depression is a peculiar type of mental condition. All seems well until the baby is born. Then the mother may unaccountably become irritable, upset by little things, morose, lose her appetite, become very tired. She is disinterested in her role as mother.

Why this occurs is not clear. It is understandable that fatigue may result from the stress of childbirth. It also has been found that in these cases the function of the thyroid, adrenals, and other hormonal glands has slowed down.

Yet it is not correct to think that childbirth is wholly responsible. It doesn't happen to all women. Other stresses may be at work. The woman's total psychological make-up may be such that childbirth is the last straw, the final stress which triggers this emotional depression.

Psychiatrists find such elements as a woman's hostility to being a woman; of disappointment at having a girl instead of a boy or vice versa; a feeling of loss of freedom — oh, many forces at work within the patient's mind.

Treatment embodies the use of thyroid in controlled dosage; ample rest and sleep; psychotherapy to help the woman understand the forces which are bothering her, often without her realizing, at first, what she resents about her life.

It may be a period of great but often vague unhappiness. The good fact is that the majority of such mothers return to normal.

Is the ability to have twins inherited? If so, wouldn't twins have to come from the woman's side of the family? Doesn't the female determine the number of children born at one time?

There can be an inherited tendency in twinning, but there is still a lot we don't know about the factors involved.

When twins are the result of the mother producing two ova, instead of only one as normal, they are called fraternal or dissimilar twins.

However, there also is evidence that the father has some influence (we don't know exactly what) over production of identical twins, or twins from one ovum. This has been noted in second marriages: A man sires twins in the first marriage, then does so again in a second marriage.

About as far as we can go is that mother doesn't get all the credit — or all the blame, depending on how you feel about having twins.

I have two sets of twins, boys 2 years old and a girl and boy, 6 months. What are the chances of another set?

My guess is that chances are good, since twinning is strongly dependent on heredity.

I am 20 and have four children. I am breast feeding the youngest, who is five months old. Is it possible to become pregnant before my period resumes?

Usually menstruation does not resume until after the baby has been weaned. However, since ovulation — and hence the possibility of pregnancy — occurs before the menstrual period, the answer is yes, you can become pregnant before your first period.

Can children of the same parents have children of three different blood types?

Yes, depending on the blood types of the parents.

Please explain the problems faced in a first pregnancy where the mother's blood is Rh negative and the father's is positive?

Possibly none at all, unless by a prior transfusion or some such means the mother has become "sensitized." For subsequent pregnancies there may (or may not) be difficulties.

The doctor obviously is already alert to the situation, and will be ready for whatever measures, if any, are needed.

My husband and I are expecting our first baby. We both have blue eyes but are hoping for a brown-eyed child. Is this possible.

Possible? Yes. Likely? No. What about the baby's grandparents and great grandparents? A few brown-eyed ones would indicate a chance. Complete lack among the ancestors means virtually no chance of a brown-eyed baby. (At birth all Caucasian babies' eyes are blue or violet; other colors appear later, if at all.)

Please settle a heated argument among four housewives. The issue is that unless a woman reaches a climax, she cannot become pregnant.

Reaching a climax has nothing to do with pregnancy.

Seven years ago I had an ectopic pregnacy and an operation. I have not been pregnant since. Does this mean I will never have children?

It's hard to say without special tests. One of the two Fallopian tubes had to be removed because of the ectopic pregnancy. Whether you can now have children depends on the condition of the other tube. If it is defective, the answer may be no. If normal, the answer may be yes.

You wrote that mothers whose babies weigh more than 9 pounds often have diabetes or may develop it. Why? I am the mother of six children who weighed from 9 pounds 3 ounces to 10 pounds 8 ounces at birth.

We don't know why. The diabetes may appear immediately or many years later.

The size of your babies is a suspicious sign but is not proof that you will have diabetes. Or you may carry the trait but not know it. Any woman having such large babies should have periodic blood sugar tests. Avoid overweight.

I plan to be married soon so would like information on birth control pills. Is it true you have to start taking them before you are married? Do you have to take them every day? Are they always effective? Is it easier to become pregnant when you stop using them? How do I go about getting them?

You will have to go to your physician to get the pills. Follow the directions he gives you, not the rule that someone else may follow. Not all the pills are alike.

In general, you take the pills daily for about three weeks, then stop for a week. Your doctor will tell you exactly which day to start and stop.

The pills appear to be the most reliable method yet devised for birth control short of total abstinence from sexual activity. For maximum safety, it is wise to take the pills for one complete cycle (a month) before being sure they are fully effective — hence start one cycle before your marriage.

In some instances, the same medication is used to regulate an irregular menstrual cycle and in that way can improve chances of pregnancy. (That was being done before the pills came to be used for contraceptive purposes.)

I have been reading about the new I.U.C.D.'s (intrauterine contraceptive devices). Are they in general use by physicians or must I go to a special clinic to obtain them?

I have been taking the pills for two years but they seem to make me tired and nervous. The I.U.C.D.'s sound ideal.

There is no perfect method of contraception except sexual abstinence, so the best advice I can offer is to choose the one that has the fewest disadvantages for you.

The present I.U.C.D.'s are updated models of devices that have been used for many centuries. Today's models may be thin steel rings, plastic spirals or circles of nylon thread.

There seems to be no agreement as to precisely why they prevent conception, but they do, even though not 100 per cent of the time.

From such reports as I have encountered, my feeling is that disadvantages outnumber advantages, but others may disagree with me.

Advantages are: No personal effort is required, no need to remember to take a pill on schedule. There are no systemic effects such as headache, nausea or bloating.

Disadvantages: The devices do not always stay in place. The expulsion rate (slipping out of position) is reported as high as 20 per cent (that is, occurring with one of five users).

There is a similar percentage of removal because of bleeding which, naturally, risks infection. There may be pelvic discomfort.

It is necessary for the woman to make fairly frequent visits to the doctor to make sure the device is in proper position.

My last child was partly strangled because the cord got wrapped around her neck, and she has brain damage. I want another child badly, but friends say I am apt to have another this same way. What are my chances compared to normal women?

The same — no problem. Please don't feel that way — as though you are different from "normal women."

After all, you had healthy children without this trouble before.

My daughter is 16, not married, and pregnant. A friend sent me some pills she got from her doctor, but I am half afraid to give them, because my daughter is between two and three months along. Will they cause any danger?

I don't know what the pills are or whether they might be harmful. But this I can say, in the hope that it will explode some decrepit and sometimes dangerous folklore: There are NO pills that will undo an established pregnancy.

How early can a doctor tell if a woman is pregnant?

With tests commonly used, pregnancy can be confirmed within 30 days or less of the time the pregnancy began. Some tests are positive within two weeks of conception, and certain hormone tests will show it within a few days.

Can abcessed teeth cause harm to both mother and unborn child?

Abcessed teeth can act as a focus of infection and produce symptoms in the mother, but I am not familiar with any effect on the baby.

I am a nursing mother. I suspect that I may be pregnant again. Will my milk supply dry up because of this?

Pregnancy has been known to suppress the milk supply — and, contrary to folklore, nursing does not prevent pregnancy. You may find on the other hand, that you DO have enough milk to continue nursing. Weigh the baby regularly to determine whether he is getting enough nourishment. If not, then start weaning him promptly.

I recently had a baby but it died two hours later. This was due to tissues in the lungs not fully developing. Do you think it might happen again?

This is one of the rare accidents of childbirth.

A baby is born without air in the lungs, so

it is turned upside down to "milk the throat," thereby removing any fluids from mouth and throat.

Room temperature often is sufficient stimulus to make the baby start breathing. If it doesn't, a sharp spank makes it cry — and that forces it to start breathing.

Sometimes this fails because of hyaline membrane disease, which is a peculiarity of the lining of the lung, especially in premature babies. Likelihood of a recurrence of this in another pregnancy is remote.

What about the pregnant woman who smokes? I am now three months along and want to know if there are any known cases of a child being mentally or physically deformed because the mother smoked. What medication is safe?

I've long thought it preferable if pregnant women didn't smoke, but I've never gotten to the point of flatly prohibiting it.

As for drugs, we have the terrible example of thalidomide. It is a good rule, particularly in early pregnancy, to take no medication except by prescription. Doctors are becoming more and more cautious in the use of any medications with which they have not had plenty of past experience. Better safe than sorry.

Smoking, if excessive, is thought to tend toward smaller babies and premature labor, and prematurity is a danger in itself although not in the sense of a deformity. Too much prematurity can, of course, be a threat to the life of the child.

What are the chances of a mother of three girls having a son? What is medical science doing now to help parents plan the sex of their children?

The ratio for all births is 1,049 boys to 1,000 girls.

In your case looking forward to a fourth baby, the statistical probability of having a boy is about 51 per cent. At any time and for any mother, the probability of having a boy (or a girl) still stays close to 50-50.

Science is trying to find some additional facts on which to proceed. We know that sex is determined by an X chromosome combining with either an X or a Y. But we do not know how Nature selects chromosomes.

There is no confirmed way to control the sex of babies. But Nature seems to do a fair job of it.

If you happen to have a FOURTH girl, you can be rather sure that some other mother is having a fourth boy. Nature at work!

I have a discharge from the vagina that seems to be getting heavier and sometimes itches. What can I do to stop it?

Various types of vaginal discharges — the general term for them is leukorrhea — are a very common type of female complaint. They may be mild, and in other cases may cause severe itching and irritation. They are not "normal."

There is no "home remedy" that will suffice. The only sound advice I can offer is to go to a gynecologist. He can determine which type of infection is present — trichomoniasis is a very common one, caused by a parasitic organism called Trichomonas vaginalis. A yeast type also is common.

Chronic infection of the cervix is a common cause also. And there are others less prevalent.

The physician, except in the most stubborn cases, can prescribe treatment to suit the type of infection.

One important word of warning: These infections can spread to the husband although they seldom bother him. When the wife is being treated, the husband should also be treated, so he won't give the infection back to her again, after she has it cleared up.

Six years ago I had surgery for breast cancer and am thankful for good health since then. For the last 18 months, however, I have been bothered by swelling in my arm. The doctor says that elevating the arm is the answer, but with a job and a family to care for, there is little time for that except when I am asleep and that is difficult. I am not complaining but have you any suggestions?

Usually such swelling occurs sooner, if at all. Scar tissue and interference with the flow of lymph in the armpit causes the trouble.

Yes, elevation of the arm is important, but good results also come from physiotherapy (baths, massage, etc.) and use of a long *elastic sleeve*.

If there is a rehabilitation center nearby, it would be worthwhile for you to seek treatment there. If not, discuss the other suggestions with your doctor and point out to him your difficulty in keeping the arm elevated.

Many women discover a breast lump during a shower or bath. In my opinion *any* lump deserves immediate diagnosis. Many are due to simple cysts. A puckering of the skin over the lump is an ominous sign.

I would rather see a lump removed, although innocent, than to wait and wonder and be too late.

Next to a lump, a discharge from the nipple is the commonest complaint related to breast disorders. The discharge may be of various types: Clear, milky, colored, bloody.

While many such discharges are due to non-malignant causes, all should be investigated — particularly bloody discharges. They may indicate cancer.

A Pap smear may be done; also mammography (X-ray examination of the breast).

If a lump is present, it should be removed for microscopic study.

This has been troubling me. If I had my tubes clipped and tied, could they untie themselves and could I become pregnant again?

There seems to be a misunderstanding of the term "tied." An ovum must pass through the Fallopian tubes in order for pregnancy to occur. When the tubes are cut and tied, the tying consists of tying a suture around the ends of each cut tube. The tubes themselves are not knotted. The severed tubes cannot reunite spontaneously. Sometimes they can be put back together surgically, but very often they can't.

What causes endometriosis and what can be done to relieve it? My menstrual periods are becoming very painful.

Endometriosis is a displacement of some of the tissue which lines the uterus. It becomes attached to the inner wall of the abdomen instead of remaining where it belongs.

When menstrual periods occur, this misplaced tissue reacts to hormonal changes, but cannot slough off easily, as it does in the uterus. It results in increasingly painful menstruation in older women — that is, in the 30's or later.

The pain stops, of course, when menstruation ends. Hormone treatment should be tried first; if that does not afford sufficient relief, then surgical removal of the ovaries stops the trouble.

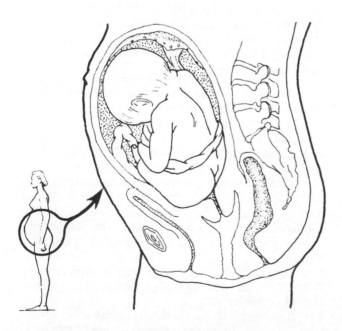

BREECH BIRTH
In four out of a hundred births, the child emerges feet first. By means of X-ray and manual examination, the doctor will know position of baby before birth begins, and will be prepared for the type of delivery he faces.

I am a recent bride. What about sexual relations during pregnancy, and during the menstrual period? This has puzzled me but everyone says it's all right.

Everyone says? Most physicians suggest ceasing relations for at least the last six weeks or so of pregnancy; under some circumstances your doctor might have other instructions. As to during the menstrual period: it is a matter of personal hygiene and esthetics.

If a woman still has her tubes and ovaries, but the uterus and cervix have been removed, is pregnancy possible?

No.

What effect does a tipped uterus have on conception?

It can, in some cases, make conception difficult or prevent it. In other cases it may not have any effect. It can be corrected surgically.

Do birth control pills cause fibroids?

No, but the pills should not be used if fibroids already exist, as they may enlarge.

I am 80 and have been wearing a pessary for several years on account of prolapse. Would an operation at my age be O.K.? I am comfortable.

If you are comfortable, and the pessary is effective and causes no irritation, why not continue as you are?

Is it safe to take a douche every night? Is it safe to use vinegar every time?

My recommendation is a flat "no" to both questions. Daily douching is not necessary for a healthy woman, and can wash away natural secretions and thus cause irritation. The best rule is to take a douche only when your doctor prescribes it for some specific medical purpose, and in that case he will also advise you what to use, and how often.

I am still a virgin. A year ago after my first year in high school I began having a whitish discharge. My mother says it is nothing, but I would like to know your opinion.

Doubtless a vaginitis, or inflammation, for which there are several extremely common causes, often from the presence of a microscopic parasite.

Have it treated before it becomes chronic.

Can a female swim during the menstrual period? Why or why not? Aren't some of the ideas about not going horseback riding or exercising a little out of date? Is there really anything one can't do at this time without harm?

As for swimming, there might be some problem involved in a sanitary pad becoming wet with contaminated water and not changed promptly. The tampon type obviates this. But other than that, there's no reason to avoid any normal physical activity. A study of college women showed that cramp was much more common among physically inactive ones, and less common among those who customarily got plenty of exercise.

Can an emotional upset cause menstruation to skip a month?

Yes. This occurs quite frequently in girls starting college or nursing school — that age bracket. The condition corrects itself ultimately.

Would the use of tampons by an unmarried woman increase the risk of cervical cancer?

No, whether a woman is single or married.

About 43 members of our club are interested in knowing the answer to this: If a woman has a partial hysterectomy, with uterus removed but ovaries left in, can normal sexual life be carried on?

Normal sexual life continues. This is true whether the hysterectomy is partial or total.

Is it possible for a woman with syphilis and without treatment to give birth to a normal baby? How long can a person have syphilis and not know it?

Unless the disease has been treated, ordinarily there will be a miscarriage, or the baby will have congenital syphilis. Even though the baby may at first seem to be normal, it may later develop some condition such as, for example, "spiking" of the teeth (Hutchinson's teeth) when they appear.

Fortunately most states demand blood tests before marriage and also blood tests during pregnancy, the earlier the better, so there is little excuse for a prospective mother not being treated before the baby is born.

How long can a person have syphilis and not know it? Quite a long time, no doubt — if they deceive themselves into ignoring symptoms.

What does D. & C. mean? Is this the same as a scraping? What symptoms would indicate that the procedure is necessary? Is it done under an anesthetic?

D. & C. means "dilation and curettage," scraping of the lining of the womb.

Yes, it is done under anesthesia.

Excessive or irregular bleeding is the principal but not the only reason for doing this. Tissue removed by the curettage is studied for any abnormality. Often, however, the D. & C. procedure alone corrects the difficulty. This is because under some circumstances tissue or material adheres to the surface and incites bleeding. Removal of the material permits a return to normal.

A D. & C. also is done after an incomplete miscarriage which may be featured by continued bleeding afterward. Essentially, the situation is much the same as described in the preceding paragraph.

A positive Pap test also is an indication that may call for a D. & C., the purpose then being to discover whether the abnormal cells found are coming from the womb above the cervix, and if so, from what area.

In other words, a D. & C. can be either diagnostic or a treatment in itself, and sometimes it is both.

If the doctor tells a woman, after a vaginal examination, that she has a large fibroid, does the diagnosis mean surgery? He didn't say fibroid tumor. Just fibroid. Can this become cancerous? He didn't sound much concerned.

A "fibroid" is a fibroid tumor — one which happens to consist of excessive fibrous tissue mixed in with other tissue.

The presence of a fibroid doesn't necessarily indicate surgery. A substantial number of women have fibroids without experiencing any trouble from them.

The uterus is a combination of muscle and special tissue which is peculiarly under control of glandular action. Because of this, it is more likely to develop tumors.

When such a tumor has been discovered, it is always wise to check periodically on its progress, if any. Sometimes a fibroid will remain the same size indefinitely for many years. If it is not causing trouble, and is not changing, there is no need for removal. And fibroids sometimes eventually subside or grow smaller at and after menopause.

My doctor advises me that I will soon have to undergo a hysterectomy.

Is it considered major surgery? Does it bring about menopause as well as end the possibility of pregnancy? What effect physically and mentally will it have on me?

Hysterectomy is removal of the uterus, and fibroids are the most frequent cause. A tumor may be so large that there is pressure on the bladder, bowel or other organs. Or, depending on its location, it may be causing excessive bleeding.

Yes, a hysterectomy is major surgery. So is removal of an appendix. However, neither should cause alarm.

Removal of the uterus prevents childbearing. But in cases requiring such surgery, the presence of the tumor already is, in most cases, sufficient to prevent pregnancy, so for practical purposes this is of no importance.

As to whether it brings on menopause, that

depends. If a woman is in her 40's and hence near menopause anyway, adjacent structures, such as tubes and ovaries, may well be removed.

Removal of the ovaries does, indeed, bring on "surgical menopause" although it is, after all, little more than a matter of speeding it up a year or two.

In younger women, the ovaries may be left in, assuming that they are healthy, show no signs of being cystic, etc. In that case, menopause will not come with the operation, but will occur at the regular time (usually about 45) when the ovaries stop secreting hormones in accustomed quantity. If, however, the ovaries are seen to be faulty, this is the best time to remove them.

Your articles on hysterectomy and the Pap test interested me very much.

Recently I had a hysterectomy as a result of a Pap test. I went to the Cancer Center because I didn't know a doctor as I've always been in perfect health.

Two biopsies were done before the operation.

It's hard to explain my feelings just now about all this. It's like a miracle, a dream. The cancer was detected so early. I'm only 30 years old. You see, I just went for this test "out of the blue." Now my doctor calls me "Mrs. Fortunate."

Your cancer might have been discovered later, and in time. Or it might have been discovered too late.

The Pap test, or "smear test" is simple, economical and painless. The doctor simply uses a small paddle to take a sample or "smear" of the mucous fluids at the cervix, or opening of the uterus or womb. Under a microscope abnormal (cancerous) cells become visible.

It is possible in this way to detect cancer in its very early stages, before it has caused a lump, bleeding or any other symptom, and before it has spread.

The cancers, at this stage, can be removed with the greatest assurance of complete cure.

The test was discovered by the late Dr. George N. Papanicolaou, who lived long enough to see it save thousands of lives.

Some gynecologists now advise women to have the test annually from the age of 30 upward; some think it might find some cancer even earlier than that, and reduce deaths from cancer of the cervix to almost zero.

What causes one breast to be larger? Does this mean cancer? How can I check for it? I am not very well-developed, so there is a noticeable difference. I am 17.

Unequal size of the breasts is not unusual. In fact, most of us, male and female, are unequal from left to right in many things. Rarely if ever do you find a face which is perfectly balanced, and photographers have had some fun showing how different most of us would look, including world famous beauties, if both sides were identical.

Studying ourselves, we find this to be true, even though nobody else notices it. So inequality in size of the breasts is nothing to be astonished about.

At 17, cancer is quite unlikely, although I'm gratified that girls are aware of the problem because that means (I hope) that they will be on guard against it later in life.

I am 53, haven't menstruated for six years, and I still get hot flashes. I had a hysterectomy a few months ago and that didn't stop them. My doctor says it isn't from menopause. If I have to put up with them, I would like to know why. What are the causes?

I have been told that no mere man has any business talking about hot flashes because he

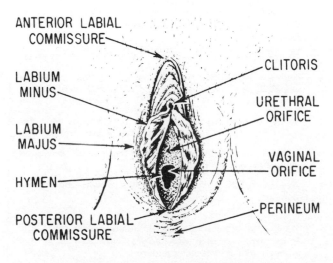

VULVA OF 18-YEAR-OLD VIRGIN

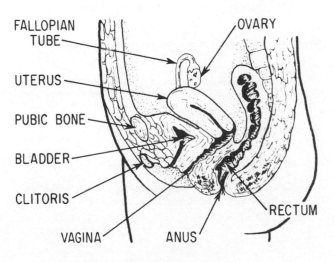

FEMALE PELVIS

doesn't experience them and therefore doesn't know what he is talking about.

With this preface of humility, I'll try to answer.

Hot flashes are a characteristic although not universal symptoms of menopause or change of life.

They are thought to be due to instability of the automatic control of blood vessels — a rush of blood through the surface blood vessels brings a sudden sensation of warmth. Hot flashes.

They are not dangerous, any more than a blush is. But they can be upsetting. They bother some women a great deal, others very little. Both intensity and duration vary widely.

This instability in blood vessel control apparently is due to the abrupt change in hormone balance which occurs at menopause. This explains the fact that giving hormones for a few months at this time helps prevent or minimize the hot flashes until the body has achieved a new equilibrium, hormonally speaking.

We do note, however, that the nervous type of woman seems to have more trouble, and it lasts longer. Hence in some cases tranquilizers or mild sedatives are very helpful, without use of hormones.

As a rule the hot flashes wane and disappear within a reasonable time but some women, and emotionally stable ones, too, report cessation when the "change" is over, only to have them recur later on. Fatigue, an emotional crisis, anxiety can trigger them, it seems. Adequate rest can be important.

In addition we know that hyperthyroidism (over-active thyroid) can be involved and that this is more common after 50 than formerly had been supposed.

Does sex activity cease after menopause? If so, I think Mother Nature is sadistic. I am 50 and haven't had a period in a year. Now that I don't have to worry about pregnancy, I am disappointed that my sex drive is gone. My husband is very virile. Can you help me?

It is quite common for the sex drive in women to increase because of the point you mentioned, no further fear of pregnancy. However, a very strong emotional element is involved. My suspicion is that somehow you got the idea implanted in your head that sex drive MIGHT decline. So it did. Knowing that the drive does NOT stop then, and knowing that Mother Nature isn't sadistic, may be all that you need.

THE NINE MONTHS OF PREGNANCY

End of Month	Mother	Baby
1	Possible nausea and vomiting. Frequent urinating at night. Sleepy in early evening. Breasts may be larger, pigmented area increased.	Embryo passed the microscopic stage, is now a visible, tiny piece of tissue.
2	Nausea and vomiting may continue. Breasts continue to enlarge, increased blood supply, bluish veins appear.	Over one inch long. Face is formed, limbs partly formed. Has definite appearance of infant.
3	Possible dietary cravings, emotional upsets. Abdomen shows signs of enlargement. Tissue at entrance to vagina is bluish.	Three inches long, weighs one ounce. Limbs, fingers, toes and ears fully formed. Sex can be distinguished. Nails begin to appear.
4	End to nausea, vomiting and sleepiness. Begins to feel unusually well, energetic, with a sense of well-being.	Eight inches long, weighs almost eight ounces. Movements can be felt, heart usually heard, bones detected by X-ray. Eyebrows and lashes formed. Skin is pinker, covered with fine hair.
5		Twelve inches long, weighs one pound, has hair on head.
6	Continues to bloom and feel well. Pink or silvery white lines, called striae, may appear on abdomen and breasts.	Fourteen inches long, weighs almost two pounds. Skin is wrinkled, and fetus looks like old man. Will usually die if born at this stage.
7		Sixteen inches long, weighs about three pounds. More fat under the skin. In male, testicles are in the scrotum.
8	Breathing may be difficult. Baby is pushing the diaphragm up, causing shortness of breath.	Eighteen inches long, weighs about five pounds, has good chance to survive if born now.
9	Increased desire to urinate may return, especially at night. Baby's kicking may cause pain. Much shifting and moving about.	Average length about twenty inches, weighs about seven pounds.
At Birth		Head is as large around as shoulders are across. Infant is less wrinkled than previously, almost smooth, and is covered with a cheeselike material.

Infant & Child Care

INFANT AND CHILD care embraces such a multiplicity of problems that it is quite impossible to try to include everything that someone will want.

This chapter, however, includes questions most often asked by readers of my newspaper column about diseases, feeding problems, behavior and so on.

I offer these generalities:

While it is necessary for a large proportion of our people to depend on the "family physician," or general practitioner, it is preferable to have a pediatrician if one is available — a specialist in child health. But the general practitioners do marvelous work, too.

The specialized Children's Hospitals in many of our cities should always be kept in mind when unusual problems develop.

Finally, I direct special attention of *everyone* to the closing article of this chapter, dealing with accidental poisoning. This is so frequent, especially around the age of 2 years, that every household which contains a child or may be visited by a child should be checked by its occupants. Common, everyday household materials cause the vast majority of poisonings.

Please tell me something about rheumatic fever in a small child. What is the treatment? What precautions should be taken afterwards? Will my young son grow out of it?

Rheumatic fever is caused by the streptococcus germ — the type which causes strep throat. It can make the child (or adult) tired, along with painful joints and tenderness of the abdomen in many cases.

But the most serious attacks inflame the mitral valve of the heart. Scar tissue forms, and the valve can become seriously damaged.

Worse yet, a child does not "grow out of" this heart damage, and he doesn't develop an immunity. He can get rheumatic fever over and over again, and in fact a patient who once has had it is more likely to get it again. And each time there is the likelihood of further damage to the heart.

Treatment basically involves antibiotics to suppress the strep germ, plus care to see that the heart is not overtaxed — it's not necessarily possible to tell immediately whether the heart is involved in a given case, so the best rule is to assume that it may be.

Precautions afterwards? Positively yes! Strep throat (let's say any sore throat) should be reported to your doctor at once. But better still, take steps to prevent any further attacks by the germ.

This, fortunately, can be done by giving regular injections (about once a month) of a long-lasting, slow-release type of penicillin.

My son is 26 months old and thus far says only a few words. He is with a mentally-retarded playmate of the same age a lot of the time. Could this have any effect on his development?

At approximately this age, the general rule-of-thumb is that a child should be able to say 10 to 12 words, and join two or three words in short sentences. But some children are faster and some slower. The degree of normal variation can be considerable.

Frankly I doubt that association with the retarded playmate has much to do with this except that there may be somewhat less incentive or competition for your son. Retardation isn't "catching."

It is more likely that, knowing about the playmate, you are extremely sensitive and concerned. Don't be. Just use normal conversation at home and your son will add to his vocabulary at his own rate.

I have been told there is a chart to estimate with a fair degree of accuracy at a certain age what a child's ultimate height will be. Could you print it?

It depends on what you mean by "a fair degree of accuracy." There isn't any entirely dependable way of predicting. A tall child is likely to be a tall adult — obviously.

The rough rule of thumb is to take a child's height at the age of three years and double it.

Charts or tables have been worked out,

averaging the results observed with hundreds of children, and while the entire chart is too long to print here, I'll give you some typical ages.

Take the child's height in inches at any of the given ages, multiply it by 100, and then divide by the corresponding figure in the chart. The answer is in inches.

AGE	BOYS	GIRLS
6 months	37.67	39.84
12 months	42.23	44.67
24 months	48.57	52.15
5 years	61.60	66.64
10 years	78.74	84.76
15 years	94.60	99.31

These figures are correct for averages, but who's average? The average is the figure which is between those who wind up shorter than the chart shows, and those who wind up taller, and that's all you can say for it.

As you can discover from the chart, at any age, girls have achieved a greater proportion of their final height much sooner than boys.

At 15, girls (again, on the average) are within a fraction of being as tall as they ever will be. But boys at that age will grow another 5½ per cent, or another three inches or so.

Heredity (quite important), nutrition, and general health (important, because it can throw off the height at various ages, and hence fool you as to what the final height will be) are factors that are hard to estimate.

And there can be some variation in the exact timing at which children go into their growing spurts. Their growth isn't steady; they spurt and slow down, spurt and slow down.

When you recently wrote about a child being born Mongoloid, I didn't know what you meant. "Webster" says: "Mongoloid, resembling, or characteristic of, the Mongols; a person having Mongoloid traits or characteristics." I can see no reason for this causing death. Would you explain?

Mongolism or "being born Mongoloid" refers, medically, to a particular type of defective child. The cause is obscure, but it is known that an extra chromosome is present — 47 instead of the normal 46.

Such a child's features (depending on the degree of the particular case) are Mongoloid in appearance: Position and angle of the eyes, thick lips, stubby fingers, and others.

Such children are mentally retarded — again, the degree of this varies. They are also of less than normal height. While this defect is not in itself a cause of death, such children have less resistance to infection; many die in infancy or childhood. Some also tend to have heart trouble. Especially with modern health care, a good many now are growing to adulthood.

When children's first teeth become so loose they can be pushed out with your finger, should that be done? Does taking loose teeth out make permanent ones grow in crooked?

When a tooth is loose, remove it. It's about ready to come out anyway and the child probably will wiggle it out with the tongue, or lose it while eating.

At that stage, removal will have no effect on the second teeth. They already are pushing up behind the first ones, and whether they are crooked depends on other factors.

My husband says he read an article stating that there was no need to warm a baby's bottles. He thinks this is true and asked me why I warmed them. I told him that anyone with common sense would. What is your opinion?

Like anything else that runs counter to tradition, the "cold bottle" idea has stirred up a storm. It was studied about five years ago by a pediatrician, Dr. J.P. Gibson. He did so because one day a young mother asked whether cold milk would hurt her baby — she'd been too tired to warm a bottle one night. To her surprise, the baby gobbled it right down.

Until then nobody had ever studied the subject. But the question came to mind: Was it any different from feeding ice cream to little ones? In his study, Dr. Gibson advised letting a bottle warm up to something like room temperature.

With very young babies, about 50 per cent accepted such a cold bottle. About 75 per cent of somewhat older babies took the cold bottles. After a week of cold milk, something like 89 or 90 per cent of the babies accepted cool or cold bottles.

All the babies showed normal weight gain, and I don't see why they shouldn't. The milk had the same food value, regardless of temperature.

Hence while it may seem reasonable to warm a baby's bottle, the evidence shows that it isn't always necessary. This doesn't mean that a cool bottle is better than a warm one. And it seems apparent that a few babies prefer it warm.

What causes a cleft (or hare) lip or palate? Is it hereditary? Can a child with no family history of it have a harelip?

It isn't always hereditary but it may be. Infections in pregnancy can cause this and other deformities. The hare lip and/or cleft palate should be corrected soon after birth.

Will you explain the PKU disease?

"PKU" stands for phenylketonuria, or the presence of phenylalanine in the urine.

The danger lies in the fact that this means that the body is not using up the phenylalanine derived from food.

In about 1930 a Norwegian chemist discovered that some retarded children had this excess of phenylalanine. The discovery was one of the important steps in preventing retardation.

Here is the picture. Phenylalanine is one of the amino acids, or "building blocks of the body," which we get from protein. It is essential. We have to have some. Yet when a child does not properly use up this amino acid, and it accumulates in the body, it can damage the brain and hence cause retardation.

This accumulation is the result of what is referred to as an "inborn error of metabolism." Some individuals are born with a defect in an enzyme which is vital in making use of that particular amino acid.

The child is born with normal intelligence, but as the phenylalanine builds up, the damage occurs. Once this has happened, it cannot be undone.

If the condition is discovered early in life, the child can be given a special diet which will include only small amounts of phenylalanine. The child then grows up without impairment of mental ability. It is, in short, one of the few types of mental retardation which we definitely know how to prevent!

How do you know when a baby has PKU?

There is a very simple test which will show when phenylalanine is appearing in the urine, which is a test for the disease.

An easy, inexpensive test! But when it means the difference between having a normal child and a retarded one which may have to spend all the rest of its life in an institution, there is no excuse for not testing every baby. In many states this test is required by law.

The doctor discovered that our eight-year-old boy's testicles are not in normal position, and that our four-year-old boy has one that is withdrawn.

Both are being given hormone shots. Since I have heard rumors that such medication can make boys effeminate, I'm doubly worried.

The doctor advises surgery if the shots don't help. I would appreciate your opinion.

This condition is known as cryptorchism or undescended testes. Hormones frequently correct it. If not, then surgery is indicated. The problem should not be neglected because testicles if left undescended can become diseased. You have some leeway to wait and see, especially with the younger boy. The surgery is usually performed between the ages of six and 12.

Your worry that the hormones might make the boys effeminate is without foundation.

My four-month-old daughter was born with a large red spot on her arm. Our family doctor says it is a collection of tiny blood vessels and will disappear when she is 4 or 5, but it seems to grow bigger and thicker every day. Should I take her to a specialist? Is it possible to have it removed?

Such a spot is called a hemangioma. I'd presume that your doctor said it "may" disappear in a few years, because many of them do.

Some don't, but they can be removed surgically, and it's a familiar operation. If the hemangioma continues to grow, consult your doctor so he can send you to a specialist.

We have been told that our 5-year-old son has cerebral palsy. Is this a permanent disorder?

Cerebral palsy is really a group of disorders, rather than a single one. It is a permanent condition. Treatment and training are possible — indeed, I hope all C.P. children get such care — but not with the hope of curing a child.

The problem is that certain portions of the nervous system have been damaged — nerve cells controlling the muscles.

In about two out of three cases, it will be the "spastic" type of cerebral palsy. The child's muscles are tense and rigid.

For most of us, the muscles relax when they are not in use. With the spastic child, two sets of muscles remain tense. When he walks, he has to overcome the resistance of muscles that should be relaxed. Such a child uses a great deal of energy to do things which for the rest of us are easy.

There are a number of kinds of cerebral palsy, and there are many degrees of it, from slight to severe. Some youngsters have trouble speaking and swallowing; others don't. They reach for something and the arm goes in an unexpected direction. A few have a tremor type — they may have good control of their muscles while at rest, but begin to shake when they are excited or when they try to do something. And there are still other variations.

Relaxing drugs, physiotherapy, patient training in how to use the muscles despite the handicap, braces, and in a few cases even surgery can help. Since cure cannot be expected, the next best thing is to teach the child how to be as efficient as he can despite his handicap, and that is what you must keep constantly in mind.

Whatever type of this disorder the child has, he needs sympathetic help from parents and doctors and therapists. He needs the courage to keep trying, and the optimism to make him realize that he can improve.

What should I do when my child has an attack of vomiting?

There are now suppositories available without prescription that work like a charm.

Severe vomiting, particularly when accompanied by diarrhea, can be quickly dangerous for an infant or small child. The loss of fluids and minerals, plus fever if it is present, can lead to acidosis, and prompt steps must be taken to alleviate the condition.

In adults, vomiting can result from various causes — appendicitis, intestinal obstruction, kidney colic, pregnancy, gall bladder disease, viral infections (often called "intestinal flu"). Naturally such other symptoms as may be present should be noted, to indicate whether the situation involves some serious underlying cause, or is a transient intestinal upset. In children, viral infection, appendicitis or intestinal obstruction are usual causes.

For the uncomplicated cases of vomiting, one of the simplest remedies, yet often highly effective, is a half teaspoon of table salt, dissolved in three ounces of water, or a bit less than half a cup.

The dose is one tablespoonful of this solution taken by mouth every 20 to 30 minutes. It can be surprisingly helpful.

Along with it, sipping carbonated drinks as ginger ale not only helps to settle the stomach but replaces fluid that has been lost. The sugar (not present in the one-calorie beverages) also affords some nutrition.

As the nausea subsides, salty broths or soups supply fluid, minerals that have been lost, and nourishment. Fluids also can be given in the form of fruit juice, or the sucking of ice chips. Candy, if tolerated, will, like the fruit juice, provide sugar to combat acidosis. (Acidosis in a child can be recognized by listlessness and fruity odor of the breath.)

Once the child can start solid foods again, crackers, toast, soft egg, apple sauce, custard, milk and juices in small amounts, but taken frequently, restore strength, nutrition and mineral and protein balance.

Our granddaughter has a stuttering problem that started when she was four. It is becoming worse. Now she is eight and self-conscious about it, and I am afraid it will affect her school work. She gets very good marks now.

About one child in 300 stutters — and for every girl who stutters, there are four boys. Why? We don't know. Many girls get over it, so that among adults the ratio is about 300 men stutterers to one woman.

Some sort of psychological stress is involved in stuttering — psychological rather than physical. Most stutterers can sing easily. Most stuttering children talk to their dolls or toys or dogs (or talk to themselves) without stuttering.

What does it mean? That the stutter is emotional! When a child is completely at ease, he doesn't stutter.

The more he stutters, the more tense he becomes, and the more tense he is, the more he stutters. Sometimes this tenseness occurs in a naturally left-handed child who is forced to write right-handed. Or a child who is teased, scolded, frightened, pushed too hard. Other cases come from tensions which are not that obvious.

Perhaps a child detects, but cannot describe, family friction. Or worried parents. Or the child is unduly sensitive to some small thing which seems very important to him, yet we don't recognize.

The best means of combatting stuttering, at the present stage of our understanding, is to help the child feel at ease. The more pressure we put on him to "stop stuttering," the harder it is to stop. Yet the same child, trying to do his best in some other endeavor, such as running, drawing pictures, doing arithmetic, or anything he feels confident that he can do, may become so interested in what he is doing that he "forgets" to stutter.

Our son started walking at about a year old, with both feet toeing inward. He is two now and still walks that way. We bought him some shoes to help him walk straight, as suggested by friends. He walked straighter and fell less. The doctor recently checked his feet and legs and said they were straight and that he didn't need special shoes.

So now he is wearing regular shoes again but with his feet turned inward, and he falls often. I am worried. Could you advise me?

It is common for toddlers to toe in — the feet are naturally flat and this position is most comfortable.

If you are still concerned, possibly an examination by an orthopedist is in order, but from what you tell me I suspect that this boy is quite normal and his feet will straighten out automatically rather soon.

Kindly advise how to get rid of pinworm in a child once and for all. He has been under a doctor's care, has taken medicine, scrubs his nails, we wash door knobs, etc., but he still becomes reinfected and it is affecting his nervous system and school work.

There is no way to do it "once and for all" except to avoid reinfection. Pinworm is not a germ. The pinworm is a parasite which thrives in the intestinal system. Very effective medications are available, including a fine "single dose" type, which will kill the pinworms in the intestine.

But a pinworm lays myriads of almost invisible eggs in the rectum, or just outside the anus. Children, by scratching themselves, or at play, or from bed clothing or garments, get the eggs on their fingers and then into their mouths. And then comes another crop of pinworms in a few weeks or months.

Others in the family also may — even without itching — be lightly infected with pinworms and thus spread more eggs.

Best rules for pinworm are:

1 — Have the whole family treated at the same time.

2 — Put great stress on washing hands after every visit to the bathroom; first thing in the morning; before every meal or snack.

3 — Try to teach a youngster to keep his fingers out of his mouth.

The only way to be rid of pinworm "once and for all" is to prevent the invisible eggs from being swallowed.

What causes croup and what can I do for it? I have tried many remedies which friends have recommended. Sometimes they work, sometimes they don't. Croup always seems to occur in the middle of the night and you can't rush out to the doctor.

Croup is a form of laryngitis. A child's larynx is small to begin with. Then infection makes the vocal cords swollen and red. There may be spasm from frequent coughing — and then you have croup.

A strep infection is the most common cause, but the viruses of the common cold and influenza are frequent, too. It is less usual these days for diphtheria to be involved. It used to be frequent.

A cold or similar respiratory infection precedes the croup. It so happens that some children never have croup in spite of colds, but when a youngster does have it, he is likely to be a repeater until he outgrows it — the age bracket is generally from two to seven years. After that croup almost invariably ceases. Perhaps it is because the larynx is larger by that time.

If you have a child who is subject to croup, watch for the first signs of a cold or similar infection. There is no way of curing a cold, but you can make sure the child doesn't become too tired or chilled, and is kept calm and comfortable.

There are all sorts of pet remedies; I happen to be a parent who went through this problem, and what worked best with my youngsters was steam with a little benzoin added.

A warm poultice on the chest often helps. Occasionally an ice collar or "cold compress" on the neck may be beneficial.

These are old-fashioned remedies, but they work, and both parents and children get more sleep.

Antibiotics have their place in keeping down infections, but they do not do any good with viruses. Your doctor will have to guide you as to when antibiotics will be of use.

Another old-fashioned remedy which still proves successful is ipecac to induce vomiting. This is unpleasant but often effective. Since too much ipecac can be dangerous, have your doctor advise in advance how much to use for a child of a given age.

My son was born with a loud heart murmur, and the doctor wrote on the chart a questionable congenital heart defect. A little later he was X-rayed but there was no evidence of an enlarged heart.

Now at 3½ months the murmur persists. However, he eats well and is gaining two pounds a month. The doctor says not to worry too much. At a year old he will have tests taken to make sure the heart is not enlarged.

The doctor says the first indication that the heart is not adequate is when the baby shows no weight gain. My only observation is that he breathes heavier than normal, and I am still apprehensive. Should I consult a heart specialist?

I must quarrel with the idea that failure to gain is the first indication of a heart that is not adequate. However, it is quite true that with serious heart trouble a child will not grow at a normal rate.

Therefore the assumption is that your baby's heart is able to meet the demands made upon it at present. The heart may, for all I can say, continue to be strong. I have no way of knowing that.

So far, your doctor has shown every sign of knowing what he is doing: He found the murmur, he had X-rays taken, he has watched the baby's rate of growth, and has told you that he wants further tests taken when the boy is a year old.

You should keep this in mind, too: Except when a heart condition is critically severe (and this case certainly does not appear to be such) more accurate studies are possible after the child is a little older.

The murmur may or may not indicate something wrong. Some murmurs disappear. In fact, a good many do.

My little daughter has been constipated from earliest infancy. The doctor said the outlet is too small and had me dilate it at home. She is now seven months old and still has this trouble, so I give her laxatives and suppositories. When she is quite a bit older will the trouble continue?

The anal opening can be too small. This is one of several possibilities. Some other disorder (such as fissures) may produce spasm and tighten it with the same result.

Your main concern now is to keep the stool soft: More water, and more laxative foods on the order of pureed prunes and applesauce.

The trouble may gradually correct itself

naturally as she grows older. If not, X-ray of the colon and other examination may be necessary to determine whether an abnormality is causing the problem.

For the present, I would not give her too much laxative medication. Rather, if water and laxative foods are not sufficient, resort to a glycerine suppository occasionally, or a small water or oil enema.

You can create a bowel cripple by fussing needlessly about trying to regulate evacuation to some particular schedule, and by overmedicating. This happens, I regret to say, to children who are physiologically normal but do not have bowel action as frequently as parents happen to think is correct.

My son had thrush mouth at the age of five weeks. The doctor gave me a prescription for him, but he still has this trouble. His mouth is just white inside. What causes it and is there a cure? Can it return?

Thrush is an infection of the mouth membrane caused by a yeast-like fungus, Candida albicans. It causes a white membrane which, if peeled away, causes bleeding.

The fungus is quite common but seems to affect principally newborn children whose nutrition is deficient, or who are not very strong.

If any question arises as to whether a case is thrush, microscopic examination of scrapings of the tissue will settle it.

One treatment which has been found to be usually effective is swabbing twice a day with one or two per cent solution of gentian violet, but I know that other treatments are used.

Yes, thrush can recur (and it also can be stubborn, too) and once you get it under control it is wise to watch for any sign of recurrence, and stop it promptly. The fungus can be present in the household environment, and can survive indefinitely in dust.

We lost a child, 3 years old, due to a brain hemorrhage from a weak blood vessel. Could this be hereditary and our future children also be affected?

It is extremely unlikely. Some fragility of blood vessels can have a hereditary aspect, but since you and your husband are healthy, it is vastly more logical to assume that this was just a tragic accident of nature, and is not likely to occur in another child.

What about braces for children's teeth? Some people tell me they're not worth the trouble and expense, and sometimes good teeth loosen and must be pulled! My dentist tells me my 9-year-old daughter and 12-year-old son both need braces, since the "bite" isn't right. I'm afraid I'll be sorry I don't take them both to an orthodontist. What do you think?

Well, first I think "some people" were completely off base and not correctly informed when they made that remark about "good teeth loosen and must be pulled." That just isn't so. Not in the way they put it.

Here are the facts, and you'll see how these people have confused things.

Straightening and aligning teeth is not an overnight process. It takes time and skill and special appliances which may be "braces" or may in some cases be rubber fittings which exert a steady pull.

In consequence, the process costs money. However, the cost is spread over some period of time. Is it worth the cost? That depends.

For others, however, the purpose is much more than good looks. If the teeth don't meet properly, we call it malocclusion — the "bite" isn't correct. This can cause a variety of problems later on — difficulty in chewing, faulty wearing-down of the teeth, crevices in which food can collect, decay, bad breath and cavities. Or throwing the jaw out of line.

BABY TEETH AND PERMANENT TEETH

Approximate time of their appearance.

BABY TEETH

1. central incisor—7½ mos.
2. lateral incisor—9 mos.
3. cuspid—18 mos.
4. first molar—14 mos.
5. second molar—24 mos.
6. second molar—20 mos.
7. first molar—15 mos.
8. cuspid—16 mos.
9. lateral incisor—7 mos.
10. central incisor—6 mos.

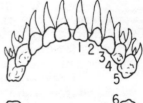
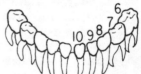

PERMANENT TEETH

1. central incisor—7-8 yrs.
2. lateral incisor—8-9 yrs.
3. cuspid—11-12 yrs.
4. first bicuspid—10-11 yrs.
5. second bicuspid—10-12 yrs.
6. first molar—6-7 yrs.
7. second molar—12-13 yrs.
8. third molar—17-21 yrs.
9. third molar—17-21 yrs.
10. second molar—11-13 yrs.
11. first molar—6-7 yrs.
12. second bicuspid—11-12 yrs.
13. first bicuspid—10-12 yrs.
14. cuspid—9-10 yrs.
15. lateral incisor—7-8 yrs.
16. central incisor—6-7 yrs.

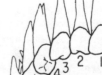
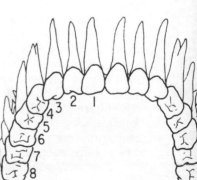
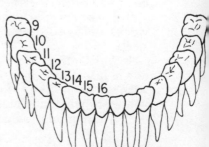

Gradually moving the teeth into proper position does not loosen them. Indeed, if you have a tooth pulled, the adjacent ones gradually (and quite naturally) will "drift" toward the open area, but do not become loose because of that.

However, in the process of straightening teeth (or even without that) it sometimes is necessary to remove a healthy tooth. This is because we sometimes inherit a jaw from one parent but teeth from the other. I'm sure you've seen this plenty of times. There isn't enough space for all the ·teeth. In such instances, it may be necessary to extract a healthy tooth in order to leave adequate room for the rest.

What should be done for convulsions? My husband had them when he was a child; then our son; now our two grandchildren.

When our son was small, the doctor said to put him in a tub of warm water, then give him aspirin and an enema and keep him warm enough to sweat.

Now the doctors say to sponge children with cool water until temperature is normal, and give aspirin. Which method is right?

Convulsions are not an illness. They are a symptom. The commonest cause in infancy is a high fever. And little ones can have a high fever quite suddenly at the onset of a cold or one of the common childhood diseases.

(There can be other causes: Low blood calcium or sugar; birth injury; brain infection; poisoning; epilepsy. If convulsions continue beyond the ages of five or six, careful search should be made for such causes.)

Why do some children have rather frequent convulsions while others have none, or few? It appears that some have more sensitive nervous systems which can be triggered into a convulsion. One study showed that in about 50 per cent of such attacks, there was a family history of others having had the same experience when young.

These convulsions, while scary for parents to watch, are brief. The first rule is to keep the youngster from hurting himself as his muscles convulse. Just wrapping him in a light blanket gives such protection.

After that, sponging with tepid (not cold) water tends to reduce the temperature. Rubbing the back with alcohol is good, too, but be sure that it isn't too cold. Use just a little alcohol at a time on the palm of your hand.

A small dose of aspirin is fine, but nothing should be given by mouth until the convulsion is over. I would not torment the child with an enema. This was advised some years ago, and I judge it was the product of an idea which once was popular, that an enema automatically helped "whatever ails you." This has long since been discredited.

My grandson recently came down with chicken pox and I advised my daughter-in-law to keep him in a dark room because some children's diseases can affect the eyes and heart. Of course I'm old-fashioned. Am I wrong in reminding a young mother of the dangers of children's diseases?

There's nothing old-fashioned about health protection. You are not wrong in advising that a child with an infectious disease be kept in and kept quiet. For one thing, it prevents spreading the disease.

There are other reasons, too, particularly relating to measles and mumps. The darkened room is for measles. The disease does not affect the eyes in a damaging sense, but it causes photophobia or abnormal sensitivity to light. Subdued light (it does not need to be a totally dark room) is more comfortable.

A more serious matter is the possibility of encephalitis or other complications from measles. Keeping the child quietly in bed lets him muster his physical resources to throw off the infection and avoid complications which can be extremely serious and even cause death.

Now that effective measles vaccine is available, this disease and its dangerous complications can be prevented — if parents will just see that their children have this vaccination.

With mumps, keeping a child quiet and in bed is for much the same reason: To prevent complications, which are most likely to affect the ovaries, testicles and pancreas.

My sister-in-law's baby always slept on his stomach. He is now seven months old. Today when she stood him up, his feet turned out. Could this be from always sleeping on his stomach?

It's quite natural for many babies to sleep on their tummies. Some do, some don't. It has no effect on the feet.

When a baby first stands up, his feet are likely to turn out. At seven months he isn't even ready to stand by himself. When he does start, he'll look — as most babies do — like a little robot, feet out, legs stiff, as he tries to keep his balance. Wait until this youngster has started walking by himself before deciding whether his feet need anything done to them.

Our 5-year-old son has hydrocele. The doctor tells us he should have an operation. Please explain it in lay terms.

Hydrocele is an accumulation of fluid in the scrotal sac, and there may be a lot or only a little. The cause is the failure of an opening into the abdominal cavity to close. A baby may be born with that flaw, or it can be caused later in life from injury.

The hydrocele (the fluid accumulation) does not damage the testicle, so sterility is not likely.

At the same time, the condition is a nuisance and it isn't going to cure itself. The fluid can be aspirated (withdrawn through a needle) but this is only temporary and it will gather again, so I would go along with your doctor's advice and have the condition taken care of surgically, once and for all, now.

My 7-month-old grandson has a very severe case of cradle-cap. He scratches his head until it bleeds. What causes this, and what do you suggest as a cure?

Cradle cap is a skin disorder which is a form of seborrheic dermatitis, which is very common among young people and even affects older ones, up to 30 years or so.

Let me spell it out. Dermatitis merely means some condition involving the skin. Seborrheic refers to the thousands of tiny glands in the skin which excrete a sort of oily or waxy substance which keeps it lubricated and supple. Too little, and the skin is dry and crackly. Too much, and the skin has other troubles. Maybe it becomes too oily. Or some of the tiny little glands become clogged and we have that frequent problem of young folks, acne or blackheads.

If, as sometimes happens, a baby or very small child has skin glands which produce more than the required amount of this oily-waxy substance, it tends to harden and create what seems to be a sort of scab. This can be irritating. It also creates a convenient place in which germs can congregate and multiply.

That's cradle cap. The scabs should be gently removed. Don't damage the skin! If a patch of the scaly stuff won't come off, leave it and take it off later, after it has become looser.

Keep the scalp scrupulously clean. Some of the oily-waxy material will wash away, instead of forming a scab. Don't try to scrub it; just wash and rinse.

When my five-year-old son is particularly upset or hurt, he cries until his breath leaves him and he passes out. This has been a problem since he was 14 months old. It doesn't happen very often but it concerns me. I don't think it is a bid for attention since he has fallen down and done the same thing while playing alone.

Breath-holding is not an unusual method youngsters use to express their displeasure. Violent crying can precede breath-holding.

The temporary cessation of breathing causes unconsciousness — and as soon as that occurs, the child relaxes, his automatic reflexes take command again, and the brief unconsciousness ends with the first breath.

Such attacks usually occur in the first couple of years, and not often after five.

One would suspect that there is some violent emotional factor in the background, maybe an overactive sense of frustration, a hidden fear of something, or the expression of extreme temper. These are possibilities and you may want to keep this in mind and perhaps have some psychiatric guidance if matters persist. That is to say, pain from a fall or whatever may trigger some pent-up emotional pressures within the child.

One report discloses that 25 per cent of children with breath-holding spells were found to have anemia. A calcium deficiency may also be present.

Children tend to outgrow breath-holding in time, but correction of anemia and/or calcium deficiency, if present, may hasten the improvement.

What is mumps? How long should a child be kept in bed with mumps?

Mumps is an acute, infectious disease caused and transmitted by a virus, in much the same way colds are spread.

It particularly attacks one or both of the parotid glands — the parotids being some of the saliva glands located at the angle of the jaw. The swelling of these glands makes that part of the neck uncomfortable. There can also be ear ache, soreness of the jaw, fever.

But other glands may also be affected at times, principally the breasts, pancreas and the reproductive glands, the testes and ovaries.

Thus, although mumps is "one of the children's diseases," and quite common, it warrants respect in case of complications. Proper treatment, however, is usually relatively simple.

This consists for the most part in keeping the child quiet so he or she conserves strength while the body is battling the virus.

This is even more true when an adult, not having had mumps as a child, catches the disease. It can make an adult quite ill. When the testes are affected, sterility can result.

It's best to keep a child in bed until the fever has subsided and the swelling has gone down. This may be several days, or a week, or perhaps two weeks in some cases, depending on whether there are any signs of complications.

My three-year-old son is pigeon-toed and has fallen arches. His right foot turns in a little more than the left. What kind of shoes should I get for him? Would an arch-support type make his feet turn in?

It isn't too unusual for children to toe in slightly; the fallen arches, however, can be serious. Some youngsters, of course, have a much flatter arch than others, without any harm resulting.

But your son may have some severe trouble shaping up unless you prevent it. Therefore I do not recommend that you do anything about shoes until you first have his feet examined thoroughly. Depending on the problem, your pediatrician may handle this, or it may prove that an orthopedist should be consulted.

Our 10-year-old grandchild has had warts over most of his fingers for the last two years. Can anything be done to get rid of these awful looking things?

Frankly, the best advice is to ignore them. They do no harm other than looking "awful."

Warts, simply an overgrowth of the skin until it forms a horny lump, apparently are caused by some as yet unidentified virus. It also appears that, for reasons unknown, some people (mostly youngsters) are more sensitive to the virus than others.

If necessary because of the appearance or uncomfortable location of a wart, it can be removed by your doctor by cautery or other means. (That does not prevent others from developing.)

Sooner or later warts have a dependable habit of disappearing no matter what you do or don't do.

My four-year-old son doesn't talk. The only thing he has ever said is "ma-ma-ma." He seems to understand everything we say, but is very stubborn and hard to make mind unless it is something he wants to do. He gets what he wants by pointing and grunting, and shakes his head for "no." What can be done to help him learn to talk?

By this age he should be talking a blue streak, of course. Or jabbering pretty well, at least. There's quite a bit of variation in youngsters so I don't believe in getting worried too soon. But I'd have the little fellow examined. There could be some defect in his speech organs that need correcting. If not, a child guidance center might be very helpful.

I have a two-year-old son. Is circumcision necessary? Why? If so when should it be done?

If the foreskin can be easily retracted and the area under it kept clean, circumcision is not necessary. However, if it is taut, and especially if there are signs of irritation, circumcision is advisable.

My daughter has been toilet trained since she was 21 months old. She is now 31 months, and has suddenly refused to use the toilet and constantly wets her pants. I have shamed, scolded and ignored her and am now at the point of spanking even though I know it does no good. She is very bright and knows she is doing wrong. Have you any advice?

It could be a psychological rebellion. But it also could be a urinary tract infection which is not uncommon in children. The first step would be to have her examined by your doctor.

WEIGHT-HEIGHT-AGE TABLE FOR BOYS BETWEEN ONE AND SIX YEARS OF AGE (WITHOUT CLOTHES)*

	AVERAGE WEIGHT IN POUNDS FOR EACH SPECIFIED AGE (Girls average about a pound less in each instance.)						
Height in inches	1 year but less than 1½	1½ years but less than 2	2 years but less than 2½	2½ years but less than 3	3 years but less than 4	4 years but less than 5	5 years but less than 6
25	15						
26	16½						
27	17½	18					
28	19	19					
29	20½	20½	20½				
30	21½	22	22	22			
31	23	23	23	23½			
32	24½	24½	24½	24½	25		
33	25	26	26	26	26		
34	27½	27	27	27½	27½	27½	
35	28½	28½	28½	28½	28½	29	
36	—	29½	30	30	30	30	30½
37	—	31	31	31½	31½	31½	32
38	—	32½	32½	32½	32½	33	33
39	—	—	34	34	34	34	34½
40	—	—	35	35	35½	35½	35½
41	—	—	—	36½	36½	37	37
42	—	—	—	38	38	38	38½
43	—	—	—	—	39½	39½	39½
44	—	—	—	—	40½	41	41
45	—	—	—	—	—	42	42½
46	—	—	—	—	—	43½	43½
47	—	—	—	—	—	45	45
48	—	—	—	—	—	—	46½
49	—	—	—	—	—	—	47½

* From 'The Child from One to Six', Children's Bureau Publication No. 30.

If nothing is wrong physically, he may, by discussing the problem with you, help figure out why the little girl is rebelling. Is there a new baby in the family? Does she feel she is not getting her share of attention? There are many possibilities.

Punishment and scolding cannot be expected to do much good, if any, and they may do some harm. At the age of five, a child is ashamed of being a bed-wetter.

Decreasing fluids for the child in the late afternoon and the evening is usually helpful.

My 7-month-old grandson, perfectly healthy except for a runny nose, died in the night of interstitial pneumonitis. Please explain how this could happen.

I can only speculate, but it is no more than fair to point out that these tragic crib deaths without warning often prove to be from lung complications.

Interstitial pneumonitis is another way of saying that widespread pneumonia developed, obviously suddenly. This can happen to children when they encounter a particularly virulent virus against which they have as yet not developed any immunity.

Such overwhelming and frightfully rapid lung infections have been proved to be the real cause of deaths once ascribed to smothering under the bedclothes.

My 19-month-old daughter has a very small appetite. The doctor says it is just a phase and that when she gets hungry she will eat.

All she wants now is milk and fruit. I have tried making her sit in her chair until she eats something, but she has sat as long as two hours and still wouldn't eat anything, so I gave that up. She eats hardly any meat or vegetables. Of course I give her vitamins, but is she eating enough to build strong bones and body?

It's just human psychology, but most mothers wonder whether children are eating enough. And doctors, who naturally see a lot of these children and their mothers, rarely find the problem worthy of worry.

Why? Because people — and that includes babies — eat when they are hungry. Of course, one must make sure that the baby is healthy. If her weight progresses within normal limits, she's getting enough to eat.

Trying to force additional food is futile and sometimes potentially harmful. With impeccable logic, any baby will take the position that "if I'm not hungry, why should I eat any more?"

It is important, of course, to see that a growing child gets the right foods. Milk is as close to being a balanced food as any we know. Fruit is a good source of some vitamins and some energy and some bulk.

To be sure, a child of 19 months should eat a certain amount of meat and vegetables. Some, however, are slow in accepting more chewable food.

But I don't condone the idea of sitting a child down in front of food and making him or her remain until it is eaten. If a child refuses to eat lunch, just take it away without making any fuss about it. No dessert. No between-meal nibbling or treats. He or she waits until the next meal.

Occasionally a child will put up quite a vociferous protest, and will sometimes stage a pretty good tear-jerking imitation of being abused. In such a case, ignore any wails and pitiful acts. Quietly stick to your guns. Pretty soon he or she will eat because of hunger.

Our young son is left-handed, but his father insists that he write right-handed. The boy's script is very poor, and he is becoming mouthy and unruly, and calm only when his father is not around.

Forcing such a child to write with his right hand makes as much sense as insisting that your husband write with HIS left hand.

The correct way is the natural way, and if a person is left-handed, he should remain so.

Forcing a child, for no good reason, to write unnaturally is one rather sure way of upsetting him psychologically and perhaps leaving him with a sense of awkwardness and uncertainty all his life.

By all means let him go back to using the left hand.

We learned two months ago that our five-year-old son has Perthes Disease. A week later he was in a brace. Our doctor said he might be in it for two to four years, and told us the bone at the hip was dead from not getting blood. Please answer the following:

1 — Could this be caused from an accident?

2 — Is there a chance of malignancy?

3 — Will the leg that is in the brace continue to grow?

4 — Is there any exercise we can use to help the blood flow back quicker?

This condition, or to give it its full name, Legg-Calve-Perthes Disease, happens to youngsters, and without fail it frightens parents. (It is due to a disorder of circulation to the bone at the hip joint.)

Your answers are:

1 — Injury of some sort is a common cause, but not necessarily a violent accident.

2 — It is not a malignant condition.

3 — The necrotic (destroyed) bone will be replaced by new bone, so the leg should grow to normal size.

4 — No, exercises won't help. The healing process is slow and there is no way to hurry it.

Naturally the brace is a nuisance, often an uncomfortable one, but taking the load off the affected bone is a vital part of the treatment. Rest and immobilization is essential.

I am 30 and the mother of three. I have had trouble with my right knee for about five years but it never bothered me enough to see a doctor until recently. The doctor X-rayed it and said I had Osgood-Schlatter's disease, and that it is common among teen-age athletes.

He suggested a cast to give the knee complete rest for six to eight weeks, but I was upset because of having to care for the children. Then he suggested a knee brace, which I am now using.

Do you think the disease could affect other bones in my legs?

True, Osgood-Schlatter's disease is usually seen in younger folks, and is thought to be the result of injury. Treatment consists of protecting the bone, by cast or brace, from further pressure until new bone grows to replace the defective area. This takes time. You and your family will have to work out the problem of providing the necessary time for the bone to rest. The outcome is usually good and there is no reason to think the ailment will spread.

Does the light from a flash bulb harm a baby's eyes, especially if he is looking right at the camera?

No. Light from the flash bulb does not contain harmfully strong rays, and it is of very brief duration.

Please write about spina bifida. How does it affect the child?

A congenital deformity, spina bifida is a failure of the bone in the lower part of the spine to unite correctly.

There are many degrees of it. Frequently it is no problem at all. In severe cases, there may be formation of cysts which in turn are subject to infection. In lesser cases a dimple in the skin, or excessive growth of hair in the lower back area can be signs.

Your doctor can tell whether the specific case is relatively mild, or is potentially serious and ought to have treatment.

FIRST AID KIT CONTENTS

Two one-inch bandages
One two-inch bandage
One one-inch adhesive tape
1 one-yard gauze
Twelve 2" x 2" sterile pads
Triangular bandage
1 scissors
Six eye pads
100 ¾" bandaids
1 box ammonia inhalants
First aid cream
Guide booklet
70% rubbing alcohol

POISON WARNINGS

I could not forgive myself if I did not include in this handbook some warning about the poisoning of children, and a word or two about the up-to-date methods of handling such cases when they occur.

1 — The greatest single type of poison is medication around the house, and the worst of all — probably because it is present in almost every household, and generally regarded as "harmless" — is ordinary aspirin. About once a week some child, somewhere, eats a handful and dies of aspirin poisoning. Many others are very ill but survive.

Reducing pills, birth control pills, grandma's heart medicine, alcohol in any form, camphorated oil — make it a rule to keep ALL household medication locked up, or where a child cannot possibly lay hands on it.

2 — Keep all household cleaners in an equally safe place — never just under the kitchen sink where a two-year-old may take a swig of detergent, window cleaner, bleach or whatnot. Anything containing caustics, especially drain cleaner, causes horrible, mutilating burns of the throat.

3 — Check your garage for weed-killers, fertilizer, paint, turpentine, paint-thinners. And remember one type of poisoning in which vomiting should NOT be induced. This involves hydrocarbons — gasoline, furniture polish, paint thinners, some cleaning fluids, kerosene, etc. Vomiting means the liquids or fumes can get into the lungs, causing a "chemical pneumonia" that can be more dangerous than the poisoning itself.

4 — Check the basement, too.

5 — Many common plants, from lily of the valley to nightshade, are poisonous, too. Best protection is to teach a child never to eat any berries, blossoms, plants or leaves.

6 — When a child is poisoned, call your doctor immediately. He may tell you what to do, or order you to get to the hospital as fast as you can.

7 — Explain WHAT the child swallowed, if you possibly can. Tell the brand name if it is some commercial product. In recent years, hundreds of poison control centers have been set up, with elaborate card catalogs of everything from shoe polish to perfume, so they can tell almost instantly what poisonous material is contained in common substances. Doctors often rely on these centers. These centers may indicate what first aid procedures to take, if any. If vomiting is to be induced, a good method is to put a heaping teaspoonful of salt in a cup of lukewarm water, stir until the salt is dissolved, and have the child drink the mixture, repeating every three or four minutes until vomiting is induced.

Common Disorders & Diseases

THIS CHAPTER deals with a considerable number of ailments. By "common," I do not mean that everyone is pretty much bound to get them — like chickenpox. But they are conditions with which almost everyone ought to be somewhat familiar — hepatitis, venereal diseases, cancer, Parkinson's Disease, diabetes, bursitis, tuberculosis, and so on.

I recommend reading the entire chapter so you will have some general idea of the various ailments. Then, as with the rest of this handbook, resort to the index when you need to refresh your memory in a particular case.

A distant relative has just found that he has tuberculosis. My family has been repeatedly exposed by eating at his home. Please tell me what to do. We have five young children. Will adding a little household bleach to water help sterilize dishes?

Yes, a bleach or detergent will help sterilize dishes, but that is a rather small part of the problem.

The greater danger is in acquiring the TB germ from personal contact. It can be carried in the invisible droplets of moisture from a cough or sneeze, or even on the breath of a person with the disease.

Now that your family already has been exposed, the point is to find out how many of you have actually picked up the germ.

The adults over 30 should have chest X-rays repeated at six-month intervals. As for younger persons, a tuberculin test (a simple skin test) is the first step. It will show whether they have actually come in contact with the germ.

Some months ago my boy had a tuberculin skin test at school and the doctor told him he had contacted the TB germ. Then he had a chest X-ray and it was negative. I don't know which is more reliable. Now I want the rest of the family to take a test, but should it be X-ray or tuberculin?

Both tests are reliable, but in different ways. The tuberculin skin test shows just one thing: That the person has come in contact with the germ. That's all.

Now if a person has NOT come in contact with the germ, then he can't have tuberculosis.

But if he HAS come in contact, then it is possible, although by no means certain, that he may develop an active case of TB. So that is why the X-ray test was given. And, as it turned out, he doesn't have an active case of TB.

Yes, it would be wise for the rest of the family to be tested.

The neurologist said I had Bell's palsy, not a stroke. How serious is this? Has anyone produced a cure for Bell's palsy?

Bell's palsy is the name assigned to what happens when something affects a branch of the facial nerve — that which controls muscles of the face. In a word, it is neuritis.

The nerves of the face are close to the surface. They cause the changes of the several facial muscles which express subtle emotions.

Bell's palsy doesn't affect all of the face, nor all of the expressions of the face, but it does paralyze the nerve branch which controls part of the face.

A drooping of the corner of the mouth and of the eyelid on the affected side of the face is the principal consequence.

It is not a serious ailment in the sense of endangering life or being painful. It isn't contagious. It is an annoyance.

A stroke is damage to some part of the brain, and the resulting paralysis depends on which part of the brain has been damaged. Bell's palsy has nothing to do with the brain and its signals. It is an interference in nerve signals at a "local station," and not at "headquarters."

Last week my husband's ankle swelled suddenly, as it had twice before. We thought it was from an old injury, but the doctor says it is gout. Can one ever be cured of it? How important is diet? Can the disease be controlled or will it worsen with age and cripple him?

Nobody is ever cured of gout, but with modern drugs it is possible to control the disease so well that patients go for years without another attack.

Gout is an inability of the system to dispose of enough uric acid, so it forms in crystals in the joints or elsewhere, and can be very painful.

It is true that too much rich food as well as alcohol can bring on an attack, but that is quite different from causing the disease.

With this type of treatment, you need have no fear that gout will turn into a crippling disease. If a patient is reasonably moderate in his eating, that is adequate. Extremely rigid diet no longer appears necessary for most gout patients.

The steroid drugs are effective for short term use with gout, but for long-term treatment a colchicine-probenecid combination is used to prevent further attacks. A new drug, allopurinol, is proving effective.

What makes my hands turn black when I put them in cold water?

From your brief description, I suspect Raynaud's Disease, which is a disorder of the nervous system's control of the tone of small blood vessels — and hence impaired circulation in the extremities. Chilling puts further burden on circulation, hence the darkness of the skin.

Nicotine has a decidedly deleterious effect on Raynaud's Disease. While you should see your physician for medication, just giving up tobacco affords marked relief.

What is sarcoid of the lung? Is there some medication for sarcoidosis?

Sarcoidosis isn't the most prevalent of diseases; still, it affects many thousands, and because not a great deal is written about it (except in technical literature) a patient is naturally confused and bewildered when he learns he has it.

Sarcoidosis has a knack of mimicking other ailments.

It can attack the lung, causing lesions which so much resemble tuberculosis that it has been called "pseudo-T.B." It can cause skin lesions which resemble cancer, which it is NOT.

Or it can look like a fungus infection. Again, it isn't, and it won't respond to anti-fungus therapy.

It can, in fact, attack almost any part of the body, causing nodes or lumpy lesions. In about two-thirds of the cases, the lymph glands will be involved, the skin in one-third, the eye, liver or spleen in about one-fifth. (It can attack in more than one part of the body at the same time.) It affects men more often than women; Negroes are somewhat more subject to sarcoid of the skin.

We don't know what causes sarcoidosis. There is a suspicion that it may be from an organism similar to the tuberculosis bacillus, but this has not been proved and may not be true. Sarcoid is not contagious or infectious.

While the disease may run its course and subside spontaneously, it also can be treated effectively with steroids (drugs of the cortisone series).

There is a skin test (Kveim test) which gives significant data in identifying sarcoid. The trouble is that this requires about four weeks to interpret the results.

Will you tell me something about emphysema?

Emphysema is a loss of elasticity of the lungs. By this I don't mean that the lungs aren't large enough. Rather, they don't get SMALL enough.

Sounds like a paradox? It's not. Some people with emphysema develop oversized chests, but they still are short of breath.

When you exhale, you expel a considerable volume of what we might call "used air." Then you inhale and replace it with an equal amount of fresh air.

But when the elasticity of the lungs is

SURGICAL TREATMENTS FOR PULMONARY TUBERCULOSIS

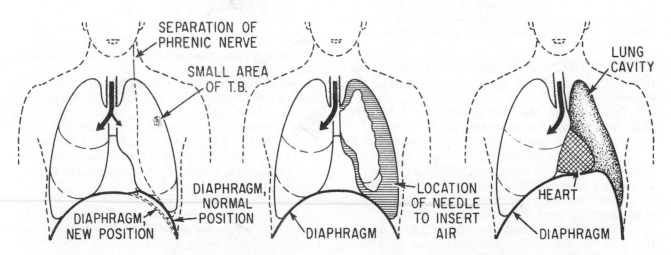

Left: Phrenic nerve is separated, immobilizing one side of diaphragm. This helps keep lung at rest while scar tissue forms. Center: Artificial pneumothorax. Air is periodically introduced into lung cavity to collapse one lung, thus completely immobilizing it temporarily. Right: Complete removal of lung. Tissue is filling gap.

lost, you no longer can exhale as much. And you can inhale only the amount you have exhaled. Too much "used air" remains in the lungs and there is less space for fresh.

Smog and other forms of air pollution, it is now believed, are a factor in emphysema. It isn't a new disease, but this is a new cause of it. But whatever the cause, you are starved for oxygen.

The answers? Some people haven't been using their lungs adequately in the first place, and learning to breathe more deeply brings into use a larger portion of the available breathing space.

Since the problem is a lack of enough fresh oxygen, it is obviously harmful to waste any of the available lung space by filling it with smoke instead of air. In a word, your doctor is going to say that the first rule is to give up smoking. He means it.

THE LUNGS

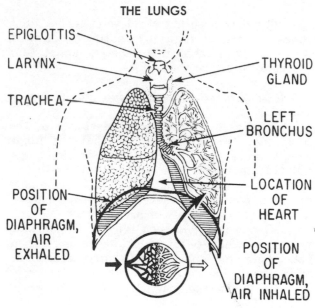

EPIGLOTTIS

LARYNX

TRACHEA

THYROID GLAND

LEFT BRONCHUS

LOCATION OF HEART

POSITION OF DIAPHRAGM, AIR EXHALED

POSITION OF DIAPHRAGM, AIR INHALED

Left: Outer surface of lung. Right: Internal structure of lung. Insert: Network of blood vessels in microscopic section of lung, showing (in black) blood before picking up oxygen, and (in white) blood containing oxygen.

Please write more about heel spurs. Do they get larger? Do they ever go away? Is surgery needed?

The lump in my heel doesn't hurt for ordinary walking but pressing on it does hurt. Should I have it removed before it gets larger?

A heel spur is not a "growth" in the ordinary sense. It is an accumulation of calcium at a point at which there has been some injury, or sometimes an infection. The calcium gathered there as part of a healing process.

Therefore, if there is no further injury, there is no reason for the heel spur to grow any larger. If there is further injury, then the spur may enlarge.

These spurs as a rule are very tiny. If you

injured your shoulder bone, for example, and a similar spur formed, you'd never notice it.

On the bottom of the heel, it's different. Your weight presses on it. You might compare it to having a very small pebble, or even a sharp grain of sand in your shoe. It feels a lot bigger than it really is.

Consequently, the best treatment for a heel spur is to find a way of keeping weight off that spot.

In severe cases, when the spur is unusually large or sharp or strategically located, surgery may be necessary.

Please answer these questions about diabetes:

1. After you start taking diabetes pills is there a chance of being able to stop them?

2. What is the difference between "high blood sugar" and "sugar in the urine"? Which is worse?

3. Does scratching (itching) go with diabetes?

4. Does diabetes affect vision? Seeing double, blur, etc.?

5. Does diabetes make you get real exhausted all at once?

6. Is it possible to have high blood sugar and not sugar in the urine?

1. Sometimes it is possible to stop taking pills later, but usually not. In some instances, insulin is necessary if the pills fail to control the diabetes.

2 and 6. Diabetes results when the body cannot use sugar properly. (The insulin produced by the pancreas is insufficient for body needs.) As the amount of sugar "gets ahead of you," the excess accumulates in the blood. That's high blood sugar. At still higher levels, sugar "spills over" through the kidneys and then appears in the urine. With proper diet, usually aided by medication, you may keep the excess sugar level low enough so it appears in the blood but not in the urine.

3. Yes, pruritus (itching) can be a symptom of diabetes. It is especially common in the female genital area. Controlling the disease helps subdue the itching.

4. Diabetes may cause visual symptoms such as you describe, triggered by variations in the blood sugar level — high to low, etc. This changes the sugar content of the eye fluid.

5. Fatigue can be a symptom of untreated or uncontrolled diabetes. Low blood sugar also can produce a sense of exhaustion or sudden weariness.

Is it possible for diabetes, controlled by diet only for many months, to be activated because of business aggravations or other suppressed mental disturbances?

Yes, such emotional upsets can cause diabetes to get out of control.

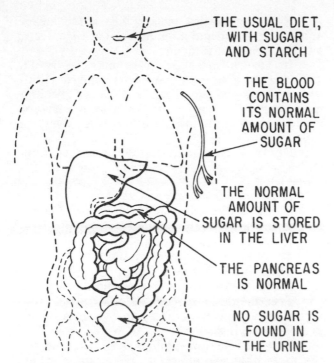

THE USUAL DIET, WITH SUGAR AND STARCH

THE BLOOD CONTAINS ITS NORMAL AMOUNT OF SUGAR

THE NORMAL AMOUNT OF SUGAR IS STORED IN THE LIVER

THE PANCREAS IS NORMAL

NO SUGAR IS FOUND IN THE URINE

The normal sugar metabolism

Does diabetes run in the family? If so, what can be done to prevent it?

Yes, diabetes can run in families, since there is a very strong hereditary element. You are particularly vulnerable if you are overweight; if you have had large babies (over 9 pounds at birth); or if you have had miscarriages.

So, if you are overweight, reduce. If you have had any of the foregoing, see your doctor for a check (urine and blood sugar tests) at least once a year. If he so elects, have a sugar tolerance test which can give an even earlier clue if diabetes is soon to start.

There isn't much, aside from weight control, that you can do to stall off diabetes. Early diagnosis and treatment usually do a great deal to prevent the complications which result from diabetes.

If a young woman marries a diabetes carrier, could she get the disease from him? Is there a cure for a diabetes carrier?

No, there is no danger at all to her. Diabetes is not a germ disease. The term "carrier," in this instance, means that a person has inherited a tendency toward the disease, and may pass on this trait to his children, but he cannot give it to anyone else.

I have diabetes and I take insulin. How often should one have a checkup?

Diabetes can vary a lot in ease of control. A brittle diabetic will show wide swings, very readily, from heavy sugar to insulin reactions.

A stable diabetic can remain sugar-free, without having insulin reactions, by taking a fixed dose of the drug.

In general, stable diabetics should consult their doctors every three or four months. It should be oftener for others. Juveniles with diabetes should be checked more frequently.

My brother, 50, has diabetes and has lost considerable weight. He takes three pills a day but his sugar count is over 250 and the doctor says if it gets over 300 he could go into a coma. That worries him but he still eats too much in the line of sweets. Should all sweets be eliminated, when taking his pills, to get the sugar count down?

Yes, I think he should eliminate sweets entirely.

Can you enlighten me on osteomyelitis? I am a woman of 56, was operated on for this bone disease 25 years ago, and it has never healed. Although there is no pain, it is discharging constantly from the opening.

Osteomyelitis is infection of bone.

Any number of things can cause it. It may be injury. A compound fracture has to be treated carefully because of this danger. Or there may be no known injury, but infection settles in the bone, migrating from a focus of infection elsewhere. Infected tonsils is a classic example. Tuberculosis is another, but the original infection may focus anywhere and be of any germ type.

In recent years, the disorder is less frequently a serious problem because of several reasons. We are more alert to subdue focal infections. We have antibiotics. Finally the importance of treating this disease early and adequately is recognized much more clearly now. These cases which linger on year after year illustrate why prompt treatment is important.

Surgery is usually necessary. In the past it was not uncommon to have multiple operations. If all of the diseased bone was not removed, the result was a chronic, smoldering site of infection and continuing drainage.

I have had neuritis for years but cannot get much relief from the many kinds of medicine I have been taking.

Neuritis is a disturbance of a nerve trunk, or perhaps more than one. Causes? Many! Injury. Inflammation or poisoning from such differing things as virus infections, focal infection of teeth or tonsils, typhoid, malaria, syphilis, diphtheria.

Poisoning can be from alcohol, lead, arsenic, phosphorus. Some of these may be contained in small amounts in medications, and certain individuals may be sensitive to them.

Alcoholic polyneuritis is found in heavy drinkers — and this can include women.

Diabetes, gout and leukemia are examples of systemic diseases which can cause neuritis.

Vitamin deficiency, especially of the B complex vitamins (as with beriberi) is another possibility.

The symptoms of neuritis are varied, too. Different degrees of pain, tingling, sharp, shooting attacks or a burning sensation; disturbances in sense of touch, temperature, sense of position or vibration. If a motor nerve is involved there may be weakness in governing the action of muscles. Or muscles may waste, or skin changes occur.

Neuritis, like rheumatism, is a word that is too loosely used by laymen to indicate a variety of pains that may not be related to it.

What is the cause of Parkinson's Disease? Would there be any symptoms in advance?

Parkinson's Disease (or Parkinsonism) is also called paralysis agitans, which means a rigidity of the muscles and tremors. It is not paralysis in the sense of being unable to move; it is a difficulty in controlling movement.

It results from a chronic disorder of certain segments of the mid-brain which have to do with control of motion, and appears to be caused by decreased blood supply to the brain — a result of hardening of the arteries.

Parkinsonism now affects an estimated 1,500,000 Americans, and as the number of older people increases, probably so will Parkinsonism.

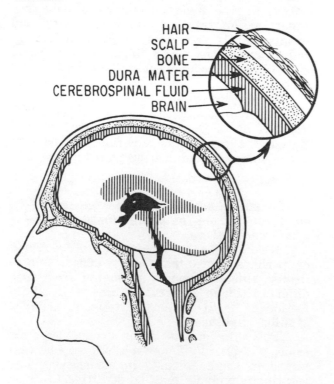

HAIR
SCALP
BONE
DURA MATER
CEREBROSPINAL FLUID
BRAIN

The number of outer coverings provide good protection for the brain, while fluid helps to absorb any shocks.

Early symptoms usually are a tremor of one hand; hand and foot movements slow up; writing becomes difficult.

In severe cases progress may be rapid. The face can acquire a blank look; muscle rigidity increases and can affect both sides; drooling may occur; the patient walks with a forward motion, as though half running and about to fall.

Dr. L. J. Dorshay, one of the outstanding authorities, emphasizes certain points of interest:

It is not hereditary.

There is no paralysis in the sense of being unable to move; rather, muscle rigidity causes awkwardness of movement.

There is no numbness or pain.

The mind is not affected.

Early treatment is important.

Treatment is aimed at alleviating this rigidity and the involuntary movements which are so annoying.

Several relaxant drugs are in use, and for the most part are effective in bringing relief, particularly if they are begun before the disease has been present too long.

In more recent years surgical treatment has been employed. It involves severing a certain area of the brain, or injecting alcohol into the critical area.

Sufferers of multiple sclerosis are not understood by the average person. Too often the staggering gait and loss of balance is viewed with suspicion and linked to drinking.

Sympathy isn't what these M.S. patients want, but understanding. I think I speak with authority because I have it.

This condition is true of some other diseases, too. For instance, a diabetic can appear to be "drunk" when he really needs urgent medical care to correct either an excess of insulin or of sugar, and his life may at stake unless somebody recognizes the real trouble. I have seen a good many such cases.

Multiple sclerosis is a baffling ailment which affects the white matter of the nervous system. This interferes with nervous control of the body. Curiously, it most often attacks young adults who otherwise are vigorous and healthy. We do not know the cause.

This degeneration can start in any of the extensive parts of the nervous system, and interference with physical activity hence can develop anywhere.

Difficulty can be followed by a period of remission in which activity appears normal.

But the condition may gradually become worse over a period of years. It is also a rather difficult disease to diagnose in its early stages. And we have no active way of treating it. In periods of severe trouble, rest is about the best we can offer.

Please discuss pleurisy. My 17-year-old daughter had it twice recently, but was relieved with medication.

The pleura is the membrane which lines the inside of the chest wall and, thus, the outside of the lungs.

When this membrane becomes inflamed, we call it pleurisy or pleuritis. Since the lungs are constantly moving, sufferers of pleurisy sometimes wish they didn't have to breathe, because it can feel like a bushel of gravel in the chest. There often is a cough. Fluid may accumulate in the pleural space, the cavity between chest wall and lungs, and sometimes needs to be drawn off.

Of course, one may have a relatively slight attack of pleurisy and not suffer too much. It can also be brief, and a combination of medications for comfort and to suppress the inflammation makes this a far less difficult ailment than it was in the days when we couldn't really do much of anything except nurse the patient and wait for Nature to achieve a cure.

Can Addison's Disease be cured?

Addison's Disease is not cured in the sense of complete recovery — like measles or pneumonia. Yet with cortisone-type drugs and adequate salt intake, it can be controlled, just as diabetes can be controlled but not cured. In many cases the presence of the tuberculosis germ (in the adrenal glands rather than in the lungs) is a causative factor. Hence the future prospects depend on controlling this germ.

Thyroid deficiency can be one of the complications in this disease.

My brother has a hernia and his doctor suggested that he go immediately to the hospital for surgery, for if he waits it will burst and he will be in real trouble.

I am worried as he refuses to do anything about it. He is wearing a hernia support and says that it is as good as going through surgery. He is 65 years old.

You undoubtedly refer to the common inguinal (or groin) hernia.

"Bursting" is not quite the term, but incarcerated. That is, the tissue in the hernia sac is pinched and the blood supply to it is greatly limited or shut off.

When this occurs, there is great pain. Immediate surgery — and I mean just that — is of utmost urgency.

If your brother chooses to tolerate the inconvenience of a truss, or support, and to run the risk of the hernia becoming incarcerated ("strangulated" is another term), that is up to him. However, if the hernia gives any pain, or a sense of tugging or pulling, he would be wise to have it repaired surgically. Trusses do not and cannot cure a hernia. All they can do is give it support.

In the case of some elderly patients, with hernias which are not too severe, it is sometimes a good gamble to use a truss and avoid an operation, but 65 is not what we consider "elderly" these days.

Is there a difference between phlebitis and thrombophlebitis? Are treatment and care the same for both? How long does it take to recuperate?

Phlebitis in inflammation of a vein, or veins.

Thrombophlebitis is both inflammation and the presence of a clot.

Treatment of the two is similar, except that with thrombophlebitis, an anticoagulant (or "blood thinner") may be used to minimize clot formation.

Rest, protection against injury to the damaged area, and measures to reduce the inflammation are the basic principles of treatment.

Time for recuperation is variable. How severe was the original attack? How good is the patient's circulation? How well does he follow orders? How sure can you be that he won't, quite by accident, bump the affected area and prolong the trouble? Does the patient have varicose veins?

What are the symptoms of a goiter? Does it impair hearing? Is there difficulty in swallowing, or seeming to be unable to get a full breath of air? Does it cause phlegm? If caught in the early stages can it be treated without surgery?

Impairment of hearing is most unlikely but the other symptoms can occur.

Goiter is an enlargement of the thyroid gland in the neck, but there are different types: It may show swelling mainly on one side, or on both; it may be nodular or smooth; it can be toxic or non-toxic; the swelling may be just in the neck, or some of it may be out of sight below the upper part of the breast bone.

The swelling can impinge on the esophagus, or gullet, giving a sense of difficulty in swallowing. It may also exert pressure on the windpipe, interfering somewhat with breathing, and causing irritation and hence phlegm in the throat.

Usually large goiters have to be removed surgically. Some types of goiter, however, can be controlled and slightly reduced in size by medication.

I recently had infectious hepatitis. My children all were given gamma globulin shots. The doctor said they would not get it, but other people say they may get a mild case.

Either is possible — but gamma globulin gives excellent temporary protection in case of an epidemic, or a case of the disease in the family.

I understand there are two types of cancer, one that is treated with X-ray, and the other with surgery. Does one kind travel faster than the other?

No, that's not quite the way it is. Actually there are many types of cancer but that isn't what dictates the type of treatment.

If a cancer is found early and can be removed totally by surgery, that's that.

Sometimes a cancer is so located that surgical removal is impossible, or is highly dangerous because of risk of damaging other organs.

In such cases, powerful, concentrated X-ray beams can destroy the cancer cells while doing much less damage to normal cells.

In some instances, advanced breast cancer being one, a combination of X-ray and hormone or other medical treatment can be far superior to either method used alone.

Please describe the technique used by doctors to examine for lumps or cancer of the breast. If my sister had not known how, she might have lost her life.

Self-examination is the first line of defense against breast cancer, and there is no adequate substitute for it. Women should be checked by a doctor from every six to 12 months, but they should examine themselves at least once a month.

Cancer organizations (American Cancer Society and others) have free pamphlets describing how to do it. Some have very effective short motion pictures to show at club or other meetings.

The first step is to stand facing a mirror and to look for any change in configuration of the breasts.

Then lie on your back. Place a folded towel or small pillow under the left shoulder. Keep the left arm down at the side. With the right hand, reach across and explore the outer half of the breast and under the arm. Don't use just finger tips. Use the entire flat area of the fingers.

This part of the examination is extremely important, as nearly half of all breast cancers start in the upper, outer quarter. Up to 15 per cent are in the second most dangerous area, the lower outer quarter.

After the outer half has been checked, raise the left arm over the head, and with the flat of the fingers explore the inner half, from breastbone to nipple.

Then move the pillow or pad to under the right shoulder, and examine the right breast with the left hand.

Not only lumps should be sought, but also any puckering or thickening, any discharge from the nipple or any restriction of movement of the breast tissues (which could indicate an attachment to the chest wall).

THE SEVEN DANGER SIGNALS OF CANCER

Everyone should memorize "the seven danger signals of cancer." None of these signals means that cancer IS present. Yet every one means that it MIGHT be starting.

Nobody should—although too many do—delay going to the doctor "because I might have cancer." Very often it turns out that the trouble is something else entirely. But when it IS cancer, the delay may mean death instead of life.

1. Any sore that does not heal.
2. A lump or thickening in the breast or elsewhere.
3. Unusual bleeding or discharge.
4. Any change in a wart or mole. (Rapid growth or change in color.)
5. Persistent indigestion or difficulty in swallowing.
6. Persistent hoarseness or cough.
7. Any change in normal bowel habits.

Is it safe to handle things belonging to a person who has open cancer on the outside of his hands and face?

Cancer is not transmissible in that way. Simple hygiene should be observed — washing your hands with soap and water after attending the patient. This, however, is not because of the cancer, but because the open areas may become infected with common germs, and you naturally want to avoid such infections.

What is a lymph gland? If one has an operation on it, what are the after-effects?

We're all familiar with the fact that we have circulation of blood. We aren't as familiar with another type of circulation: Lymph, which carries away various waste products and, in particular, disposes of the by-products of infection.

The lymph, a useful, gradually-moving fluid, follows the many little lymph ducts of the body, finally reaching a lymph gland or node, which filters out the undesirable materials which then are carried by the blood stream to the kidneys for disposal.

If you have a badly infected tooth, lymph glands in the neck may swell because they are overloaded with the task of disposing of the poison. Or with a badly infected hand there may be streaks moving up the arm — a dangerous sign meaning that "blood poisoning" is starting. What we really see is an excessive flow through the lymph ducts.

Infectious mononucleosis is noted for causing the lymph glands to swell. German measles is characterized by swelling of the glands in the back of the neck. And so on and on.

Some diseases attack the glands themselves. The tuberculosis germ is one. Cancer is another.

When one (or more) of the many lymph glands kick up a storm, a doctor wants to know why. If he sees a case of bad tonsils, connected with a swollen neck gland, he doesn't have to puzzle over the connection. It's obvious.

But when the cause is NOT readily apparent, he does (and should) begin to wonder. The gland itself can, and in many circumstances should, be removed and sent to the laboratory for microscopic examination, to find out what ails it — a germ, and which germ, or some other condition.

Removal of the gland, or part of it, for study, is no serious matter. We have lots of glands. It's a lesser thing than, for example, removal of tonsils. There are no after-effects.

Please explain the term, idiopathic grand mal epilepsy, in words understandable to a layman.

Epilepsy is a "convulsant disorder." That is, the parts of the brain which control muscular activity are affected. Involuntarily you find the muscles going into an abrupt tightening or paralysis or "convulsion."

There are two principal forms of this, the "grand mal," or severe convulsion which may last for several minutes. The patient will lose consciousness, may thrash about, bite his tongue.

The other common form is the "petit mal," which may occur very frequently in some cases, sometimes many times a day. But the attacks are mild and very brief. Often they amount to no more than a momentary pause between words or in the middle of a word, after which the person goes right on talking as though nothing had happened.

If the cause of the epilepsy is known, an injury of some sort, it is called traumatic. If no such injury can be ascertained, the case is called idiopathic.

Hence idiopathic grand mal epilepsy means a convulsant disorder, cause not known, with convulsions of a severe form.

The majority of such cases can be treated with harmless drugs which prevent most and sometimes virtually all of the attacks.

Are rheumatic fever and St. Vitus Dance the same? Do they both affect the heart in the same way?

Rheumatic fever — an inflammatory attack caused by a streptococcus infection — sometimes results in St. Vitus Dance or Huntington's chorea, which is another name for it. (The jittering usually disappears as the patient grows older.)

Rheumatic fever also very frequently attacks the heart. The valves become inflamed, and as the inflamed areas heal, scar tissue remains and interferes with their proper opening and closing. This heart damage is the serious aftermath of some cases of rheumatic fever.

My husband has been a heavy drinker for years. All at once he started to swell. His lips almost doubled. His face swelled and got red.

The doctor said it was cirrhosis of the liver, gave him a prescription and told him to eat meat, some sweets, very little fat, and to drink no liquor at all.

My husband stayed on the diet for two months and looked 10 years younger. Now he has started to drink again and won't remain on his diet. What is usually the length of time a person can live under such circumstances?

Cirrhosis means that the liver has been damaged. The damaged parts of it have been replaced by other tissue which cannot do the complicated tasks the liver must perform.

It used to be thought that alcohol was the sole cause of cirrhosis. This is not entirely true. Faulty nutrition plus some other factors (metabolic disorders, certain toxic factors, and perhaps others) are involved.

A heavy, steady drinker, however, very often is NOT careful to eat properly. Thus drinking also plays an indirect part in causing cirrhosis.

Once the cirrhosis has begun, then drinking exerts a very heavy burden on the liver, and the disease progresses rapidly.

There is little in the line of medicine that will provide much help. Cirrhosis cannot be cured! What is necessary is to make things as easy as possible for the damaged liver. This means proper diet and complete avoidance of alcohol.

Your husband was frightened enough in the beginning to follow instructions, and you saw the result. He looked years younger. What it amounted to was that he relieved his liver of the strain of faulty diet and alcohol.

But as soon as your husband began to feel better, he either decided (*wrongly*) that he was cured, or didn't realize that his diet and no alcohol were the reasons for his improvement.

Such patients, and there are too many of them, are the despair of doctors and are their own worst enemies. It is impossible to say how long a patient can live under such circumstances. It depends on how much damage already has been done to the liver.

But unless he goes back to his diet and cuts out alcohol completely, he will be sick again just about as quickly as he gained — and he will get steadily worse.

Is hepatitis catching? Does it recur later in life? What effect will it have on sex life? Does it resemble venereal disease in any way? A young man of 18 has it. The doctor has placed great stress on cleanliness and rest, but no other comment.

There are two types of hepatitis (liver infection). One is "serum hepatitis," in which the virus enters the blood stream via a blood transfusion or unsterile needles.

The more familiar type is infectious hepatitis, which is transmitted either by direct contact with a person having the disease, or by way of contaminated food or water. That is why contaminated clam or oyster beds are closed by the authorities.

Swimming in contaminated water, or acquiring the virus on the hands, and getting it into the digestive tract by eating without first washing the hands, are other ways hepatitis can spread.

The basis of treatment is to see that the patient gets plenty of rest and a good diet, adequate in protein and carbohydrate, and with some, but not too much, fat. Alcohol must be avoided completely as it puts added burden on the liver. Keep in mind that hepatitis is a liver disease.

The patient feels weary, often has headaches, and may suffer from nausea, loss of appetite and fever. Even though he does not feel like eating, he should be coaxed to do so, perhaps by frequent, small meals, as good nutrition is vital to rebuild the damaged liver.

Hepatitis does not affect sex life (once the attack is past) and has nothing to do with venereal disease.

Only rarely is hepatitis fatal if proper care is given, but it may require six to eight weeks for recovery, and sometimes longer for the patient to get over feeling listless and tired.

It is possible to have the disease again, but only from a new infection. The original case will not recur.

What causes varicose veins? How can they be prevented?

The underlying cause of varicose veins is a weakness of the veins (usually in the legs) plus anything which contributes to congestion of those veins.

Veins in the legs are under a greater strain because blood has to be lifted back to the heart, a distance of several feet.

At intervals these veins have one-way "flutter valves." When the heart beats, blood is pumped upward. Between beats, the valves close automatically, so blood cannot flow back down.

When one of these valves weakens or fails, it puts added pressure on the vein below it. Presently the whole vein is under the pressure of supporting a column of blood which moves sluggishly at best.

Then you have a varicose vein.

Best way of minimizing the danger of varicose veins is to avoid anything that restricts circulation — avoid round garters, tight girdles or other garments. (Pregnancy, because of pressure on veins in the pelvic area, can contribute to varicose veins.)

Standing still for long periods is bad for varicose veins — but walking, since it helps circulation, helps *prevent* them.

Support hosiery or elastic bandages, by supporting the muscles and veins, helps relieve the discomfort of varicose veins but does not "cure" them. The same is true of sitting periodically with the feet and legs elevated.

Only cure is removing the veins, one way or another, and thus forcing other veins to take over the work.

Sometimes smaller veins can be sclerosed or "dried up" by injections, but this is not always permanent.

The sure treatment is by surgery — either ligating (tying off) the swollen veins, or "stripping" them, which means making small incisions above and below, and then drawing out the veins lengthwise. Those particular veins then are gone for good — although it is possible that other veins will subsequently become varicose. Being overweight is a contributory factor.

I have a rash and ulcers around both ankles, which refuse to clear up. The doctor suggests an operation for varicose veins. Would this help?

With varicose ulcers which refuse to heal because your circulation is impaired, an operation for the varicose veins is about the only thing that can be expected to help.

I have recently heard of "painless hemorrhoidectomy." Of course I am not naive enough to believe that it is actually painless, but is there a newly developed method of surgery or treatment immediately afterward that lessens the discomfort? Some years ago I heard of people who suffered a great deal of pain following this surgery.

It isn't the operation that hurts, since it it done under anesthesia. It is the period afterward. The area is naturally tender. I am as doubtful as you are that it can be painless. That just isn't reasonable.

But the painfulness has been very considerably reduced. The after-care is of the greatest importance. This involves gentle dilation of the rectal canal to prevent adhesions and excessive scar formation.

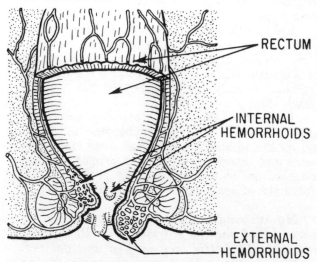

Distinction between internal and external hemorrhoids.

If adhesions and heavy scar formation are allowed to occur, it is an invitation to permanent discomfort instead of a return to natural function after a relatively short period of soreness.

My husband has pain and stiffness in his right elbow, and two doctors have diagnosed it as tendonitis. One suggested X-ray treatment and the other cortisone.

My husband finally consented to having a cortisone shot, which helped him only temporarily. Should he try the X-ray treatment, or more cortisone?

He isn't having anything done now because he believes his condition is chronic and he "must learn to live with it."

Cortisone is very effective in many of these cases. However, more than one injection may be required. If one shot afforded temporary relief, that's a good sign.

Heat and salicylates (aspirin) also are very effective.

True, tendonitis (inflammation of a tendon) might be slow to cure, but I can't agree that it necessarily is chronic or something you "have to learn to live with" until a reasonable amount of treatment has been obtained.

I am a 14-year-old girl who wants to know more about venereal disease. I have read about it in the library but don't understand why it apparently happens only to unmarried people. I asked my mother and she wouldn't tell me.

Understanding of venereal disease by young people your age is extremely important, and the book which gave you the idea that it "happens only to unmarried people" did you a disservice.

The two principal venereal diseases are syphilis and gonorrhea. Both are caused by germs. Both are spread almost invariably by sexual contact. One gets the disease by such contact with a person who has the disease — whether married or not.

Compare these diseases with tuberculosis. The TB germ happens to flourish best in the warm, moist environment of the lungs. Therefore it is spread primarily by people who have the disease and scatter the germs by coughing or sneezing. If the germs are soon breathed in by another person — before the germs dry out and die — the disease can be transmitted to the other person.

In like fashion, the venereal disease germs, if conveyed directly from the sexual organs of one person to those of another, can transmit the diseases readily.

Venereal disease can be cleared up readily with proper antibiotics, if treated promptly. Untreated, gonorrhea can cause sterility, or cause babies to be blind.

Syphilis is worse. At first it may appear to cause no real trouble, but over the years it can resemble or contribute to all sorts of diseases, including heart disease, arthritis, neuritis, brain damage.

The best defense against getting a venereal disease is to avoid being sexually promiscuous. The person who has sexual relations with a number of partners is pretty likely to become diseased, because some of the various partners may be promiscuous, too.

Second-best defense is to develop a high degree of suspicion. Be checked by a doctor after any such contact. "V.D." is extremely prevalent among young people, perhaps partly because young people are tending to be more sexually promiscuous, and because they are gullible and just can't believe that "that nice boy" or "that sweet girl" could possibly have a venereal disease.

Gonorrhea is easily recognized by a boy or man because of the thick discharge which develops a few days after exposure. The discharge in a girl or woman sometimes is not as heavy, but if a discharge develops approximately 7 days after a sexual contact, it is a highly suspicious sign and a doctor should be consulted.

Syphilis is not as easy for the individual to recognize. There is a small, painless "sore" at the point the infection occurs. It can disappear in a week. There may be other signs later, chiefly a skin eruption. But syphilis, unlike gonorrhea, can be diagnosed readily by a blood test. (That is the blood test which most states require before marriage.)

Can a baby be born with a venereal disease?

Yes, but only if the mother has the disease and it has not been adequately treated.

THE TEN LEADING CAUSES OF DEATH

1900	Deaths Per 100,000
Pneumonia	304
Tuberculosis	280
Diarrhea and enteritis	183
Nephritis	161
Heart disease	128
Accidents	87
Apoplexy	81
Cancer	67
Ill-defined and unknown	65
Diseases of early infancy	60

1967	
Heart disease	453
Cancer	218
Vascular lesions of central nervous system	74
Influenza and pneumonia	38
Accidents	34
Cirrhosis of liver	34
Certain diseases of early infancy	27
Diabetes mellitus	22
General arteriosclerosis	16
Congenital malformations	10

Can syphilis be transmitted by kissing? Would it show up in a blood test later?

Yes, it can be transmitted that way, especially if there is a cut or break in the skin. Yes, a blood test will show it later, certainly within a few weeks.

What is bursitis? How long does it stay? Is there any way to ease the pain?

There are small fluid-filled sacs which Nature put around joints as a sort of cushion, to let tendons ride easily. Such a sac is a bursa.

Because of injury or too much continued pressure, a bursa can become inflamed and sore. Sometimes too much fluid then gathers in the bursa. More pain and swelling.

Bursitis (inflamed bursa) goes under many names: "Housmaid's knee," when it develops from prolonged pressure from kneeling; "tennis elbow" from strain on that joint; "chauffeur's elbow" from the pressure of resting the arm in a certain position on the ledge of a car window.

How long an attack lasts is rather unpredictable. Some untreated cases become chronic. Some are cleared up in a matter of a few days, but one should be careful not to abuse the joint afterward.

There isn't much you can do by yourself except to rest the irritated joint. If an arm or shoulder is involved, a sling may be the best thing for it. Hot wet compresses may be very helpful.

Your doctor, however, has a number of things he can do for it. A simple pain reliever and rest may be enough in some cases. Injections of various medications, the steroid hormones (cortisone) being very helpful, often

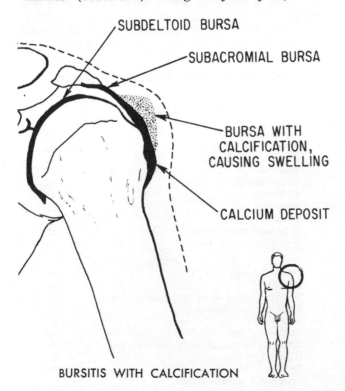

SUBDELTOID BURSA

SUBACROMIAL BURSA

BURSA WITH CALCIFICATION, CAUSING SWELLING

CALCIUM DEPOSIT

BURSITIS WITH CALCIFICATION

bring prompt relief, after which rest lets Nature do its repair work.

If the bursa is greatly swollen, withdrawing excess fluid by means of a surgical needle is an accepted procedure. Occasionally surgery is required.

What is Grave's disease? Has a cure been found for it?

Grave's disease is a severe form of hyperthyroidism (overactive thyroid). It features such symptoms as rapid heart beat, nervousness, prominence of the eyeballs.

Yes, indeed, there is effective treatment. In some instances antithyroid drugs slow down the gland's activity to a suitable rate. In other cases radioactive iodine does the job. In still others, surgical removal of part of the gland is preferable.

I was hospitalized for acute myositis and the only help given me was diathermy. The soreness and pain keep coming back. What causes myositis? Weather or diet?

Myositis means muscle (from myo) inflammation (from the itis part of the term).

Something has irritated the muscle fibers and the cause of this inflammation is the important question, as opposed to ordinary myalgia, or incidental muscle strain as from temporary lameness from too much exercise.

Heat is, by and large, the best means of easing the pain; hence the diathermy. Like so many of our ailments, myositis may "cure itself," meaning that the body automatically tries to correct what is wrong. If we can do something further to help the process along — fine! The diathermy is one thing. Rest is another.

But in a severe case it is important to look for such other things as may underlie the trouble. Arthritis, bursitis, infection, rheumatic fever, trichinosis are the most likely ones.

Myositis is what we call a non-specific disease. It doesn't attack some particular organ. Rather, it can involve muscle tissues in different areas. If the back muscles are affected it can be called lumbago.

My 20-month-old son fell on our puppy. The dog bit him under the eye, leaving three small breaks in the skin.

The child had had his tetanus booster shot only three months before, but the doctor still insisted on giving another shot and two prescriptions for medicine. Was this tetanus shot necessary so soon after his booster?

The shot was necessary for complete safety. True, the little fellow might not have gotten tetanus (lockjaw) anyway, but I certainly favor being safe rather than sorry. The prescriptions, I have no doubt, were for medication to protect against any other infection which might have been present.

Food Fads, Fallacies & Facts

I T IS HARD to think of a phase of everyday life which in recent years has been more beset by fads and notions than food. Many people pursue various "health food diets" with what seems to be almost religious zeal.

"Health food stores" are common, and advertising and sale of "food supplements" has become a big business, with claims that it is necessary to use someone's "supplements" of vitamins and minerals if you are to remain healthy.

From my observation, I cannot say that these products are harmful, but they run into money, whereas the average person can get all the vitamins and minerals he needs or can use just by eating a simple but well-balanced diet.

The body needs protein, carbohydrate and some fat; it needs a variety of vitamins; it needs certain minerals, many of them in such tiny quantities that they are known as "trace elements."

Considerable calcium is needed, both for strong bones and as an integral item in repairing tissue injuries. It is plentiful in dairy products as well as in green leafy vegetables and other foods.

Iodine is the one element which, in some parts of the world, is difficult to find in food. The almost universal availability of iodized salt has taken care of that. Seafoods contain it, and rapid transportation of such foods is another helpful factor.

For the other minerals, meat, fruit and vegetables will provide them in abundance.

Eating a balanced diet becomes for most healthy people a matter of habit. They don't keep a list of what they eat each week. They just acquire a habit of eating certain things every day (or almost every day) and of eating other things every day or two.

In this part of the world, most people get considerably more fat than they need. Appetite will take care of our getting enough other "energy" foods — starches and sugar in addition to fats.

Please discuss plateaus that occur while dieting. Hitting them has been my bugaboo after losing about 30 pounds. Sometimes I will go several weeks before an additional loss.

Most reducing, probably all reducing, involves these plateaus. You don't lose weight consistently or in a straight line.

In the beginning, the losses, and plateaus, are close together and you don't notice the pattern. Later you do.

Why does this happen? Well, as you use up excess fat you also lose the amount of water which is bound to the fat cells. During the process, water is produced by the "burning" or consumption of the fat. So you have additional water to get out of your system.

The "crash diet," which is supposed to shed so many pounds in a week or two, prohibits salt, since it tends to hold water. You lose water rapidly when you give up salt. Hence the quickie diet seems to work like a charm for a short time — until you've gotten rid of excess fluid in your system. After that it suddenly doesn't work as well, and besides, when you go back to normal eating, you go back to salt too, and you regain the large amount of water and the very little bit of real weight that you lost.

When you stick with a low-calorie diet, after a time you use up excess fat (or some of it, anyway). You don't have as much flesh that has to be nourished and kept warm. So, actually, you need a somewhat different caloric intake — not quite as much.

If you are still overweight, when you hit

these plateaus you can keep on losing.

All of the foregoing factors are among the reasons why I take a dim view of "crash diets," but I have seen very excellent results from slow, sane and comfortable reducing programs.

A year ago I started using artificial sweeteners instead of sugar in my coffee. I drink a lot of coffee, so this made quite a difference in calories and helped me stabilize my weight.

Recently a pharmacist told me these sweeteners, saccharin and the cyclamates, had produced cancer in laboratory animals and that I should avoid them. Another said that if they produced cancer, then a lot of diabetics would have cancer. Can you ease my mind?

A fantastic number of scare stories have been circulated about the artificial sweeteners, none of them founded on fact to the best of my knowledge.

Saccharin has been in use for a good many years now, and the cyclamates for somewhat less, but still long enough to indicate that they can be used without harm.

The Food and Drug Administration has had these sweeteners under virtually constant observation. If any dangerous consequences were found, you can be certain that regulations would be promptly forthcoming. To date they have not.

The only unpleasant side effect of which I am aware is that in large quantities they can, in some individuals, cause a tendency toward diarrhea.

We recently had a water softener installed. Now our friends and neighbors have informed us that this device takes away certain minerals and vitamins which are necessary to the body. What is your opinion?

My opinion is that your "helpful" friends and neighbors ought to mind their own business, and learn the facts before they try to worry you with nonsense.

There are no vitamins in water, whether hard or soft.

There are minerals in hard water. That's what makes the water "hard." But they are not in a form which can be used by the body.

Softening, by various processes, involves substituting sodium for the calcium and magnesium in the hard water.

The one thing to watch out for, with softened water, is this: People on a low-salt (low sodium) diet should avoid softened water because of the sodium it contains. It is not, however, harmful to the rest of us.

Is there any way to get rid of "stretch marks" after losing 40 pounds? Can one prevent them?

There's no way to get rid of them, but the color gradually fades. They are not a result of losing weight, but of having gained it — the skin fibers were broken due to stretching from excess fat. Some people are much more likely to have this trouble than others. The only preventive is avoiding excess weight. Cosmetics will cover up the marks.

My mother recently set out some frozen chicken broth, let it thaw completely, then changed her mind and put it back in the freezer to use some other time.

I tried to explain that the refrozen broth would not be safe but she only argued that she does this with frozen foods all the time and nothing happens. What are the facts?

Regardless of what she thinks, she IS running a risk. It may be that nothing has happened. Or something may have happened but she didn't realize why. You are quite right in saying that thawing and refreezing food can be dangerous.

Freezing can prevent germs from multiplying, yet many germs merely hibernate and become active again when temperature rises. Each thawing — and subsequently until the food is solidly frozen clear through again — allows that much more time for germs to increase.

With repeated thawing and refreezing, food can, indeed, spoil. It spoils a little at a time, but it is still spoilage.

Most commercial frozen foods carry a warning not to thaw and then refreeze. This warning is given because there's a reason!

Periodically we read about a meal or picnic at which people are taken ill with "ptomaine" or food poisoning. In most cases this is traced to food that was allowed to stand — and germs had time to multiply. It happens most readily in warm weather but it can happen any time.

The best rule is to use frozen foods the first time they are thawed. Standing for a reasonable length of time between the thawing and cooking is all right — let's say up to four hours. But definitely don't thaw and refreeze.

By the way, hasn't your mother ever encountered meat, particularly chicken, that has been thawed and refrozen? The surface gets a sort of silvery appearance, and it often feels wet and slippery as it thaws again. What causes this? Bacteria have been active during the thawed period.

Can beef broth cooked with carrots and served every day to a child cause a yellowish tinge on the palms?

Yes. This condition is called carotenemia. The coloring in yellow vegetables is carotene, which the body converts into Vitamin A.

Some of this is necessary, but eating more than is needed can cause a yellowish tinge which, however, disappears if such vegetables are withheld.

CONSUMER—BEWARE!

How did old wives' tales begin? How do modern health fads (kin to the old wives' tales) begin?

A noted nutritionist, Dr. Dena C. Cederquist, of Michigan State University, says that food fads often are based on this type of reasoning:

"Of all persons killed in automobile accidents last year, 98 per cent had eaten white bread or flour on the day they died."

That's the kind of logic the food faddists use. She goes on:

"If you tell me that you eat wheat germ for breakfast and that it makes you feel wonderful, I can't really argue the point with you because I don't know how you feel. But I can conduct tests under controlled conditions and find out what kind of nutritional value the germ has.

"The food faddists capitalize on our inability to be absolute, by telling half-truths that lead the public to believe its food supply is not adequate."

She is right. Without prohibitive amounts of testing, we can't pin down the absolute amount needed by any individual — the amount of Vitamin D, for example.

But we CAN figure out an amount that will provide a margin of safety for everyone. Going beyond that amount serves no useful purpose. Going too far beyond, and even an otherwise useful or necessary vitamin or mineral can be harmful. Yet the food fads hang on, today's version of old wives' tales.

Some of those old notions must have come about from similarly fallacious arguments. A deformed baby was born — and, seeking an explanation, yet without facts, somebody said, "I remember now. The mother ate a lot of strawberries last summer." (Or whatever happened to have been noticed.)

I can't imagine where the idea that fish is "brain food" came from, or that wine is a "blood builder." It isn't.

The frequent nonsense about "harm" from cooking in aluminum dishes isn't hard to trace — and this hokum keeps coming up often enough so that I am repeatedly asked about it. It's a fiction invented by peddlers trying to sell stainless steel or some other kind of cookingware to people who already have aluminum.

The aluminum pans, of course, are perfectly safe.

So some of the old tales (old and new versions) are the product of ignorance and others are invented because someone hopes to profit by spreading misinformation. Don't be taken in by either kind.

Please explain botulism. Will any certain processes used in home canning prevent it?

Botulism is an acute, rare and dangerous food poisoning caused by one particular germ called Clostridium botulinum.

Unlike most germs, this is one which does not require air or oxygen for growth — quite the reverse. Hence if it happens to be trapped in an enclosed food container it can continue to multiply, and unless canned properly, the germ will grow, producing a fatal type of toxin.

Cooking food for 30 minutes at 176 degrees also will kill the toxin and germ.

Are the eating patterns or mannerisms of youngsters inherited? Our three-year-old son shows active interest in everything except eating. When my wife and I discussed this with other parents, one of them said emphatically that he had inherited this behavior from relative X. Your opinion will be appreciated.

Parents can't do much to influence a child's interest in food — and maybe that's just as well. Whatever you do, you don't stand much chance of solving the problem except to raise further rebellion and your own blood pressure.

Most children eat because they are hungry. For the first two years their growth is rapid. Then, as the initial spurt subsides, they just don't need as much food. Children know this instinctively, but it's hard for parents to recognize it.

At the age of six or thereabouts another spurt of growth begins. We're all familiar with the later pre-adolescent and adolescent youngsters who become bottomless pits. It's natural.

So the first explanation for the child who doesn't eat is that he isn't hungry. The other common reasons are family discord; putting so much pressure on the child to eat that he automatically turns stubborn about it; illness; or poor eating habits, which includes between-meals snacks, especially candy and sweets.

Eating habits are not inherited. They are copied.

See that meals are balanced, and that mealtime is harmonious.

A friend claims alcohol has food value, whereas I say that it has no vitamins or minerals — only calories or units of heat.

Yes, alcohol has food value. You are right that it has no vitamins and no minerals but does have calories. However, calories represent food value. Too many calories make you fat. A drink of straight whiskey can mean 80 or more calories. Cocktails and highballs can be higher, and some of the fancy drinks with sweet mixes can be even more.

That's why some people keep gaining on "reducing diets." They forget to keep track of their drinks.

The heavy drinker who goes on a week-long bender doesn't eat because alcohol gives him enough calories — food value or nourishment — to destroy his appetite.

The same would be true if you ate nothing but sugar: No vitamins, no protein, no minerals. A week-long candy binge would be very harmful to the health, too.

Could you explain why in the morning I weigh 110 pounds, and maybe 111 or 112 in the afternoon or evening?

Easily. Take athletes, such as football players, either in a game or in practice. They lose five pounds quite readily and some even more. Most of this is in loss of moisture. Sweat. By the next day they have gained all of it back.

A pound or two is easily explainable in terms of moisture alone. You expel a little moisture every time you breathe. You can see this when people breathe on their glasses to clean them. Let's say you breathe 3,000 times or more while asleep. It mounts up into ounces of moisture.

Then at breakfast and lunch you not only eat, but you drink coffee, milk, water. You are constantly gaining or losing a little.

That's why, for people who keep track of their weight, we suggest weighing at the same time each day, preferably the first thing in the morning.

My husband is a thin diabetic. He is on insulin and a 2,200 calorie diet. Even with exchange lists, his food is monotonous. Where can I get additional information? There is no trained dietitian nearby.

With some culinary imagination, you can create variety and still not violate dietary rules. True, you can't suddenly decide to have six hamburgers for supper without pouring excess calories into the meal.

And anyway, the diabetic who is on a rigid diet, and balancing his food with insulin, has to keep that balance stable. Too much food, and sugar starts to accumulate in his system. Too little, and the insulin, not used up, can be dangerous, too.

So, I would say, the hardest thing about being a controlled diabetic may be the necessity for living a regular life and eating balanced meals. You can't go on "binges" of eating or anything else.

However, except for that, there's nothing either difficult or awful about a diabetic diet. However, there are certain restrictions. In this case, the 2,200-calorie limitation bars the occasional excesses that the rest of us indulge with impunity (more or less), but it's not too bad a total figure for a man who doesn't do heavy physical labor.

Within the calorie limit, most of us could be fed a "diabetic diet" and never notice it.

Seasoning, different ways of cooking, and substitution within the rules can afford endless variations: Cabbage for lettuce, a radish or two (5 or 10 calories), celery, endive, Chinese cabbage, watercress — there are all sorts of salad variations. Ditto for vegetables. Ditto for fruits. Ditto for rye, whole wheat, white, graham or other breads. Ditto for substitution of different kinds of meat, fish or other seafoods.

If you have a dietitian within telephone distance, it helps, but not everybody does. I suggest that you subscribe to a periodical named "The Forecast," published by the American Diabetes Association, 1 East 45th Street, New York 17, N. Y. It carries interesting menus and variations of diet in each issue, and you gradually absorb from it a lot of ideas, all physiologically sound, for making the "diabetic diet" tasty and varied.

I understand that Vitamin C taken in quantity is a good way to ward off colds. Besides orange juice and a vitamin-mineral capsule each day, I am taking a 250 mg. Vitamin C pill daily. Will this be harmful to me?

There isn't any way to ward off colds except to keep your general health good, and avoid (if there's any way to do so!) the scores of viruses which cause colds.

In consequence all sorts of notions have sprung up for preventing colds. Vitamin C is one of them.

If you truly lack Vitamin C, taking more of it will help you. Once you have enough, excess amounts won't help. However, taking it won't hurt you (except financially) since the body readily excretes any Vitamin C above its normal needs.

I have heard that excess Vitamin D, if taken over a long period, can be detrimental to adults. What would be considered excessive, and what sort of troubles can be caused?

Yes, it's possible to get too much Vitamin D, although nobody is likely to do so unless for no valid reason he starts taking supplemental portions in excessive amount.

An excessive amount depends upon the individual. In general, it would be over 50,000 units a day, although in some instances it may be as little as 15,000.

Excessive Vitamin D mobilizes calcium and phosphorus from the bones. This leads to fatigue, weakness, nausea, and possibly encourages formation of kidney stones.

Rarely does an adult need large doses of Vitamin D, since ample amounts are obtained from ordinary foods and from normal exposure to sunlight.

Children, it is true, particularly infants, may benefit from moderate Vitamin D supplements, which is why a few drops of halibut or codliver oil may be added to formulas, but the average daily requirement for a growing child is only about 400 units.

Will Vitamin E, the wheat germ kind, help my husband's arthritis? I read in an ad about a person who claimed to be cured in six months. Would there be any harm in his taking it? He doesn't eat lettuce or cereal or green vegetables, but virtually lives on potatoes, meat and cottage cheese.

If Vitamin E would improve arthritis I'd say so. So would thousands of other doctors. I see no harm in taking it, however. No special diet will cure arthritis, but your husband should eat some green and yellow vegetables and fruits. (The cottage cheese is a good source of calcium, so I don't mention milk in his diet.)

When I was 18 I weighed 245 pounds. At 24 I joined TOPS (Take Off Pounds Sensibly). I am now 27 and weigh 145. I am 5 feet 8.

Can anything be done for my flabby upper arms, hips and thighs? I have exercised faithfully for three years but have noted little improvement.

I congratulate you on taking off 100 pounds in three years (and I pay my respects to TOPS, an excellent organization) but you can't expect flabbiness from that much reduction to disappear very quickly.

Exercise will tone up the muscles, a very necessary part of your program, but remember that the skin and other tissues were greatly stretched when you had that excess 100 pounds.

There is no quick way to "unstretch" them. If too unsightly, you may resort to plastic surgery — but please keep trying exercise.

I was taught that after squeezing fresh oranges, the vitamins are lost if the juice is not used in 15 minutes. Is this true? Others do not agree with me.

Vitamin C is lost gradually through exposure to air, as well as just by standing. I suppose there would be a little loss in 15 minutes, but not much.

I am 40 and the mother of two grown children. I am slowly putting on weight even though my diet doesn't change from 1,000 calories a day. That's right — I eat one meal and watch the calories.

I consume lots of no-cal soft drinks but always feel full and bloated even if I have only one of them. I thought that as long as I'm not eating, I'd lose weight by drinking these, but I don't at all.

I feel as though all my bodily processes run at a very slow pace. I am a housewife and don't do any extra exercise. Can you help?

Here are two or three thoughts that may help. As to the 1,000 calories a day, I think you'd do better to spread them among three meals. Studies have shown that more fat is deposited from one large meal than from three or four small ones, although the total calories are the same. Eat a good breakfast. This could be quite a factor starting the day actively, and perhaps change your feeling of your bodily processes running "at a very slow pace."

I'm generally inclined to take folks' calculations of the calories they consume with some reservations — not that people aren't telling the truth as they see it, but sometimes they are mistaken.

They count one potato at so many calories; or one slice of bread, or one serving of peas, or one lean chop, yet the size (and the calories) can vary 50 to 200 per cent, from your potato, to my potato, to his potato.

It's also easy to forget small nibbles — tasting the soup, or eating a "teeny-weeny bit of candy," or drinking a glass of wine because it would be impolite to refuse.

If you actually ingest 1,000 calories a day, or more or less than that, you are still slowly gaining — so you are eating more than you use up. It is unusual (although not impossible) for people to reduce successfully without exercise. I'd suggest exercise for you. It needn't be fancy. A brisk hour of walking — and I mean brisk — is good. Or make it bowling, calisthenics, or chopping wood. It's all exercise.

The bloated feeling may come from the carbonation, the bubbles, in which case unsweetened tea, coffee or plain water may avoid the trouble. But brisk exercise may also solve this problem.

Besides everything else, if I were you I'd have my doctor check on metabolism. A sluggish thyroid can make you feel as though you are living in slow motion.

Please give me a diet for cholesterol.

I won't specify any special "cholesterol diet" because I don't think it is either needed or helpful. Some very simple precautions will do everything that can be done about cholesterol, unless your condition is such that your doctor needs to give you special medication.

Cholesterol, a fatty material, is always present in the blood. It belongs there. If we ate foods which contained no cholesterol at all, our body would still create it. Even rabbits, existing entirely on vegetable foods, have cholesterol.

The danger isn't in having cholesterol, but in what happens to it later. As our arteries harden, cholesterol is part of the conglomeration of material which attaches itself to the inner walls of the arteries, thickening them.

It has been suspected that if the amount of cholesterol in the blood could be lowered, maybe our arteries would stay healthy longer. This, however, is an assumption and not necessarily a fact. Experiments along this line show that some people with high cholesterol have good arteries, and some with low cholesterol have poor ones. This raises a question: Is some other fat, or some other condition, the really important key?

We know that people who are overweight have more trouble with their arteries and their hearts. Therefore my belief is that the more practical approach is to take care of our weight and let the cholesterol take care of itself.

We are two girls, aged 15, who weigh 140 pounds and we know it is too much. We have cut carbohydrates and fats completely out of our menus, but our parents force us to eat them for a "balanced diet." If we keep on eating potatoes, bread and cake, how can we lose weight?

Overweight is not entirely a matter of what you eat, it's also a matter of how much you eat. Your parents evidently do not realize that almost all foods contain some carbohydrate, and that's another point to consider.

If you girls get plenty of protein (lean meat, eggs, fish, dairy products) and dutifully eat your vegetables and fruit and juice, and drink a couple of glasses of skim milk a day, you will have a balanced diet. (You will get enough fat that way, too. Americans on the average eat twice as much fat as they really need.)

Can't you make a bargain with your parents? Have cereal for breakfast every day, skip cake or other desserts entirely, eat some potato, which is a good nutritious food, and it won't be fattening provided it isn't fried, slathered with butter, or covered with gravy. Say a baked potato with very little butter or margarine.

You can be perfectly healthy and still control your weight, and your parents ought to be happy. The only point that worries me is this: Some people, without any good reason, confuse plumpness with health. Maybe your parents do. Actually, you girls are on the right track.

I am taking diet pills and avoiding all foods like bread, cookies, potatoes, etc. However, I have been constipated, and have been taking laxatives. Do you think the problem is from the pills or the diet? Should I continue the laxatives?

This is a matter of what you consider constipation.

This is a rather common complaint among dieters, until the facts become clear to them. If you eat less, and have less food residue to dispose of, obviously your bowels will not (and cannot) move as plentifully as they did before. Thus what some people regard as constipation isn't really that at all.

What's your opinion of crash diets when people go into the hospital and consume only coffee, tea, bouillon and vitamins? Even under a doctor's care, isn't this dangerous? The dieters lose from 10 to 12 pounds a week.

That sort of regimen is not what I call a crash diet. It's controlled starvation!

To me, a crash diet is a quickie type that lets you lose enough in a week so that you can fit into a snug dress for Susie's wedding. Nearly 100 per cent of the time, such a crash dieter then regains the lost weight by going right back to former eating habits.

People who go to a hospital and reduce calorie intake to almost nothing are in a somewhat different category.

They are usually extremely obese and have been unable to stop eating — even though they are so heavy that it is an extreme menace to their health.

After a few days of starvation, they lose their appetites and do not suffer hunger pangs. They are under regular tests and continuous observation, and if their body chemistry becomes harmfully deranged, it can be corrected. With such watchfulness, this method is not dangerous, particularly when supervised by someone skilled in such a form of reducing. The diet ordinarily does not last more than about 10 days.

Doubtless people who are only moderately overweight could, if they cared to pay the price, resort to these hospital starvation programs from time to time. But don't you think it is better to learn how to keep your weight down, instead of having it fluctuate and incidentally, alternately stretch and unstretch the skin?

The fundamental part of any reducing program is — or certainly ought to be — to teach a person how to avoid getting fat again.

Recently I changed to decaffeinized coffee (my own idea, not doctor's orders) and began getting bad headaches. At first I blamed it on sinus and the weather. Now I have gone back to regular coffee (5 to 6 cups a day) and the headaches are gone. Could there be any connection?

Yes, it's possible. Caffein in suitable amounts is a valuable drug for headaches and is used in many remedies. There is no objection to coffee in moderation.

You wrote not long ago that too much coffee is bad.

Pappy turned 90 on Jan. 8. His quota is 20 to 30 cups of coffee daily — with cream and sugar. He starts off at 5 a.m., and the last cometh at 9 p.m., his bedtime. When he hits the sack the house could burn down and he wouldn't know it.

So — how much coffee is too much coffee?

You're exaggerating a bit. But I'll give you a straight answer. People have different tolerances. One cup of coffee is too much for some; one cup isn't enough for others.

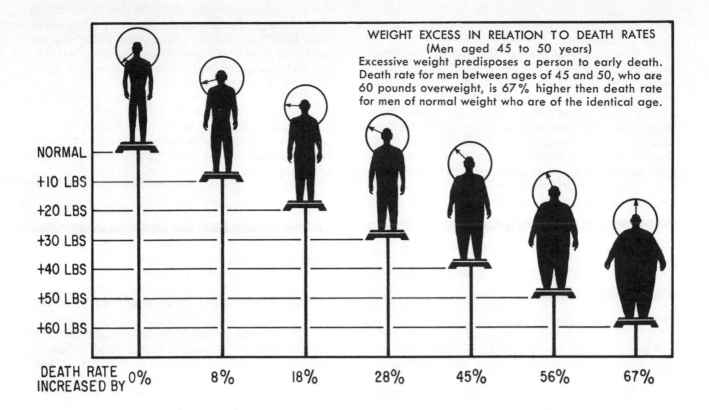

WEIGHT EXCESS IN RELATION TO DEATH RATES
(Men aged 45 to 50 years)
Excessive weight predisposes a person to early death. Death rate for men between ages of 45 and 50, who are 60 pounds overweight, is 67% higher then death rate for men of normal weight who are of the identical age.

NORMAL
+10 LBS
+20 LBS
+30 LBS
+40 LBS
+50 LBS
+60 LBS

DEATH RATE INCREASED BY 0%   8%   18%   28%   45%   56%   67%

If I run into somebody who complains that he has the jitters and his heart skips a beat, and he has to get up six times a night to go to the bathroom, then I say, "Well, let's cut down on the coffee and tea."

But if such symptoms are NOT present, I wouldn't think of cutting off anybody's coffee. But neither would I say that because some friend's Pappy thrives on coffee that everybody should follow suit.

Does coffee affect hardening of the arteries? My former doctor told me not to drink coffee, cola or carbonated beverages. He moved away. My present doctor says he doesn't think they will hurt me.

None of these drinks would have any particular effect on arterial hardening. However, caffein (whether in coffee or colas) can quicken heart rate, cause nervousness and sometimes "extra" heart beats.

I am 19 and weigh the correct amount for my height, but I have what would be called a big stomach. Whether my weight goes up or down I still seem to keep my belly.
I have been told to take daily exercises. What types do you suggest?

The tummy is, after all, a natural spot for fat to accumulate.

Check on your posture. If you sag, the stomach will bulge.

Any exercises that tone the muscles of abdomen, waist and hips are beneficial. Here are some simple ones:

Bend at the hips, forward, back, sideways. Work at it! Easy bending doesn't do much good. Bend until you can't go any farther.

Lie flat on your back. Raise one leg, then the other. Then both together. Try holding them for a few seconds just an inch or so off the floor. That really puts strain on the abdominal muscles.

Lie on your back, then pump your legs in rotary fashion, as though riding a bicycle. (This is an old stand-by for women who have just had babies.)

Do push-ups. They strengthen the abdominal as well as other muscles.

"Spot reducing" is not easy — that is, in just one place without reducing total weight.

The exercises I have outlined will burn up some of the stomach fat, but the principal benefit will be in toning the muscles.

I have always understood that milk builds strong bones, but now I have heard that too much of it leaves calcium deposits.

After all these centuries, it doesn't seem to me that milk should need any defense, but so many letters like this one continue to come in, perhaps we'd better try to set such ideas at rest.

It is true that milk provides calcium, and calcium is a vital ingredient of strong bones. If you don't get enough calcium from milk, you have to get it from some other source or the bones will suffer.

Milk, however, is the easiest and surest means of getting it. This is a problem that Nature neatly worked out. Animals from ass to zebra suckle their young on milk. Calcium, naturally, isn't all that milk contains, but all milk is rich in it.

But there is a whopping difference between calcium "deposits" and calcium which normally makes up our bones, teeth and some other tissues.

If we get too much calcium, or at any rate, more than we need, the body simply discharges the excess, just as it does with most of the minerals which we need in varying amounts. The excess does not accumulate as calcium deposits.

Rather, calcium deposits are created only in response to some damage — injury, or infection.

Restricting milk will not alter or prevent them. Too much milk does not cause them.

Which is best after a meal, to rest, or to take a walk?

A short rest is preferable followed by a walk or some type of exercise.

The body changes the blood flow depending on needs at any particular time. After you eat, blood flow is diverted so more of it goes to the digestive area.

With exercise, the muscles are competing for a greater share of blood flow.

So that's why a short rest is better after a meal. That's also the reason for not swimming for an hour or two after eating — so competition by various parts of the body for increased circulation won't occur, with a consequent risk of muscular cramps.

My husband has gout and is on a purine-free diet. Where can I get menus or recipes?

Not "purine-free," but "low purine." Avoiding all purines would be virtually impossible.

Anyway, you don't need recipes or menus; just avoid the high-purine foods. These include the "organ" or "gland" meats — sweetbreads, liver, kidneys, heart; the legumes, such as peas and beans; and herring and anchovies. Go easy on red meats. Poultry, most fish, boiled or smoked ham, lamb and shellfish (crabs, oysters, lobsters) have much lower purine content.

Evidence is mounting that diet is much less important in gout. Some caution in diet is helpful, but proper drug treatment to prevent excess accumulation of uric acid in the system, is bringing excellent results.

What is Vitamin K? And what about the advantages or disadvantages of taking a small dose a day for blood clotting?

Vitamin K has been called the coagulation vitamin.

It is helpful in making the blood clot, and thus stop bleeding, in certain cases, and not effective in others. For example, it is not effec-

tive if basically the bleeding is due to cirrhosis of the liver. On the other hand, if anticoagulants have been given, or for some other reason the blood does not have enough platelets (special clotting particles) to control bleeding, then Vitamin K is very good indeed.

Thus it is a rather complicated problem to know when Vitamin K should be used and when it shouldn't. A small dose (one a day, for example) can be very valuable if the patient is otherwise subject to bleeding because of special drugs, or some deficiency in the blood.

Let your doctor decide whether you need Vitamin K, and how much.

I enjoy potatoes, but some people say they have no food value, and are merely fattening. What about this Irish potato?

It's time somebody came to the defense of the lowly, healthful potato. Irish, Idaho, Maine or Michigan — it's still a potato and it's still good.

The "some people" you quote are slandering the potato. Of course it has food value. In fact, there is no food which is "merely fattening." True, some have more calories than others, but one thing only is fattening: That is eating more than you need, more than you use up in the form of energy and body-repair.

A potato has a little more than one-third of the calories of the same weight in beefsteak — 1,090 calories for an average pound of beef, and 375 calories for a pound of average potatoes.

The danger of potatoes, from the reducing standpoint, is that some folks insist on having them mashed and swimming in butter, or fried, or drenched in gravy. This adds relatively enormous amounts of calories.

What effect do diet pills have on the body? My doctor has prescribed them for about two years, off and on. Lately I have had headaches. I feel nervous at times and my hands shake. I am only 23.

As I've said many times before, "diet pills" have certain risks and side effects; and should never be taken except under a doctor's supervision.

I add a second rule: Remember that it is up to you to notify your doctor if the pills bother you.

The mere fact that he has prescribed pills does not automatically mean that he will know if or when they begin to bother you. No two patients are exactly alike, and they won't respond identically.

Hence reducing pills still have to be used with reasonable caution.

"Nerves" and the various manifestations of nervousness are the foremost problem. The result may be jitters, restlessness, difficulty in sleeping, or other such consequences.

Heart, Circulation & the Blood

THE HEART and circulation belong together — the cardiovascular system. They are, obviously, closely bound up together. Indeed, the most common type of heart disease is a circulatory matter, interference with circulation of the blood to the heart system itself.

I lay particular emphasis on this type of heart disease in this chapter because of the need for impressing upon folks the simple but essential methods of maintaining strong hearts. Keeping one's weight at a proper level, and regular, although not necessarily strenuous, exercise are two matters which anyone can do for himself — and the results excel anything a pill can do for you.

Various matters pertaining to the blood are included at the end of this chapter, pretty much arbitrarily. This seemed as good a place as any to put them. Here again, however, I urge readers to make use of the index, which will be the easiest way to find many items which do not fit automatically into a familiar category.

What is hypertensive cardiovascular disease? I have high blood pressure, hardening of the arteries, and get nervous in crowds, stores and even in my own home when company is present.

Hypertensive cardiovascular disease is another way of saying that high blood pressure (hypertension) is affecting your heart (cardio) and blood vessel (vascular) system.

Hypertension may be a confusing word because tension means different things. Applied to the bloodstream, tension means it is under greater pressure than normal.

But when we use tension alone, we usually think of it as meaning emotional pressure. It is possible (although not particularly likely) for a person to be emotionally calm yet have hypertension in the sense of high blood pressure.

In general, the tense, worried individual is more likely to have high blood pressure because the nervous tension is reflected in his physical condition.

The doctor told me my blood pressure was a little high. What can I do to lower it to normal?

For the patient who still wants to do something for pressure that is only "a little high," the most useful suggestion are these:

1 — If you are a tense, high-strung individual, ease up.

2 — If you are overweight, reduce.

3 — If you are worried about something, either resolve the problem or make up your mind that it isn't worth all that worry. One way or the other, get rid of it.

Worrying about your blood pressure is a fruitless pastime that just makes it worse.

What is congestive heart failure and how serious would it be in a woman of 65 who has not had a heart attack as yet and hopes to avoid one?

A heart attack means that the organ's muscle is damaged by some of the circulation to it being cut off by a clot or similar obstruction. It is the muscle which suffers — and naturally that is serious.

Congestive heart failure is a different thing. Instead of being the result of a sudden attack, it develops gradually, and from more than one possible cause.

A typical condition involves damage to one of the valves in the heart. While the heart beats as strongly as ever, the faulty valve does not let it function as effectively. So the heart has to work harder to accomplish the same amount of blood circulation.

The heart gradually tires from the strain. The seriousness depends on the degree of congestion.

Tests show that a man of 51 is afflicted with heart disease and arteriosclerosis obliterans in the lower extremities.

His legs are very weak and constantly painful. Is this disease curable or can arteries in the legs be replaced with plastic tubes? If so, can the patient use his legs normally? I have also been told that nerves in the legs could be cut to relieve the severe pain. But wouldn't this leave the patient without use of his legs?

Arteriosclerosis obliterans is a severe type of hardening of the arteries. Circulation is greatly impaired and this causes the weakness and pain.

Possibility of surgical help depends on the location of the narrowed segments of arteries. This can be determined in an arteriogram (special X-ray of the arteries).

If one of the larger arteries in the thigh or above is the site of the principal clogging, then surgery may be considered to insert a section of plastic, or in some other way (depending on circumstances) let blood flow more freely past the clogged point. This will not interfere with use of the legs. Rather, it will improve their condition.

If the principal difficulty is in the smaller vessels of the lower leg, then this procedure cannot be done successfully.

The nerve operation you mentioned is called a sympathectomy, which involves severing a special segment of nerves which control the arterial tone. That is, the operation permits greater dilation of the smaller arteries in the affected region, thus increasing circulation through them.

My husband was recently hospitalized for chest pains which the doctor called "arteriosclerotic heart disease — myocardial anoxia."

Would you explain what this means? His blood pressure was normal at the time of the attack. Should he have some kind of medication in case the pains come on suddenly? I worry myself sick from the time he leaves the house until he returns.

The first part — arteriosclerotic heart disease — means that blood vessels carrying blood to the heart muscle have become hardened and narrowed, so they do not carry as much blood to the important heart muscle.

The second term, myocardial anoxia, defines the condition a little further. "Myocardial" again refers to the heart muscle, and "anoxia" means that it is not getting enough oxygen. Not enough circulation, hence, not enough oxygen.

Read the following article for information on how this condition is managed, and the article on angina pectoris, for the pain.

What is the difference between a heart attack and heart failure? A doctor told a 75-year-old woman who was worried about a heart attack, "You have a bad heart. You don't have to worry about a heart attack, but if your heart continues to overwork, it will go into heart failure."

This woman's husband refused to take her condition seriously although she has been doctoring for five years and spends most of the day in bed.

Let's compare the heart to a water pump which is operated by an electric motor.

The heart muscle is the "motor." If you cut off the current to the motor — blow a fuse, or

HEART GLOSSARY

Angina pectoris —The chest pain from coronary insufficiency.

Aorta —The main artery conducting blood from the heart to the rest of the body—including the heart muscle.

Arrhythmia —Irregular (heart beat).

Atherosclerosis —Hardening of inner lining of arteries ("hardening of the arteries").

Arteriosclerosis —Hardening of outer wall of arteries.

Auricle or Atrium —One of the two upper chambers.

Cardiac —Adjective meaning "of the heart," or related to the heart.

Coronary insufficiency —The heart is unable to pump the normal amount of blood, so the patient tires too quickly, may develop leg cramps while walking, may develop chest and heart pain.

Coronary occlusion —Closing off some part of the artery which furnishes blood to the heart muscle.

Coronary infarction —The same thing—specifically, a lack of circulation to part of the heart muscle, causing part of the muscle to die and be replaced with scar tissue.

Coronary thrombosis —Also the same, a "thrombus" (usually a clot) shutting off the circulation.

Fibrillation —The heart quivers instead of consolidating its energy into a regular heart beat.

Heart attack —General term for all of the above. Also called "a coronary."

Heart failure —Same as insufficiency.

Mitral valve —One of the series of valves between the various heart chambers. This is the one most frequently damaged.

Tachycardia —Episodes of rapid heart beat.

Ventricle —One of the two lower chambers of the heart doing the most work.

burn out the brushes, or whatever — the pump stops. So does the flow of water.

That's a "heart attack." Clogging of an artery has shut off the blood supply (or part of it) to the heart muscle.

A very severe heart attack can, of course, be fatal. Lesser ones are not.

More than three-quarters of persons who have had heart attacks return in time to their usual jobs.

A heart attack is sudden — just as shutting off the electricity that runs the water pump, is sudden.

Heart failure is quite a different matter. Let's compare it to the washers or valves in a pump becoming worn and leaky. (Actually, other conditions can be at fault, either in the heart or in the pump.)

Anyway, the "pump" rather than the "motor" is affected. A leaky valve means that less fluid (water, or blood, depending on which simile you have in mind) is pumped with each stroke, or each heartbeat. So the pump has to work harder to maintain the same flow.

That is "heart failure."

Heart failure, unlike a heart attack, is not sudden. It develops gradually, becoming worse and worse. Nobody lives forever, of course, but the person with "heart failure," or a defective heart, can live for many years if he takes the trouble to keep his heart from having to work needlessly hard.

Please write about the heart ailment, angina pectoris. What causes it, how serious is it, and what are its symptoms?

How careful does one have to be to prevent attacks?

That's a bigger order than you may have thought. Angina pectoris is featured by severe pain in the mid-chest region — tightness, burning, fullness, or a sense of pressure there. It may also radiate to neck, shoulder and arms.

Indeed, it resembles the feeling of a heart attack in many cases; yet it can occur without an electrocardiogram showing any sign of abnormality.

Or again the angina may be accompanied by known heart disorders. You see, therefore, that angina pectoris is not a single disease; it can, with the same apparent symptoms, come from a variety of causes.

The simplest to understand is a narrowing of the arteries which serve the heart muscle. If the muscle is not getting enough circulation to match the labor demanded of it, the result is pain. It resembles an acute muscular spasm or cramp anywhere else.

As you might easily guess, too much heart strain can bring on an attack. This need not mean vigorous or prolonged activity, but only an amount which exceeds the ability of the heart to fulfill its functions with adequate ease. For one person this may mean walking up a flight of stairs, or strolling several blocks. For another a walk of half a block may trigger an attack. Likewise, since digesting our food draws blood to that area, a heavy meal can start an attack, and a person often may have to learn how much he can eat at a sitting without suffering.

Exertion also adds up. A heavy meal, plus some walking, plus perhaps going up stairs, or carrying a burden — all of these together amount to more strain than if the heart had been allowed to rest between efforts.

Other physical conditions may play a role. High or low thyroid activity, anemia, and disorders of the aorta are known to cause or contribute to many cases. Angina is relatively common among people with diabetes. And in some cases no physical reason for the attacks can be found at all. This, as you may well imagine, is the subject of some intense research.

The most effective relief for angina is placing a nitroglycerin tablet under the tongue. It gives sufficient lift, even though temporary, so that the pain ceases and the heart catches up to adequate power. The effect of the tablet, however, is brief.

Fortunately there is no particular limit to the number which can be taken safely. Neither do they lose their effect from repeated use.

If the blood cholesterol is high, reduction of it by diet and medication sometimes reduces the pain.

THE HEART IN RELATION TO THE LUNGS

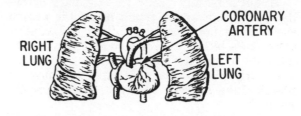

SCHEME OF BLOOD CIRCULATION THROUGH THE HEART

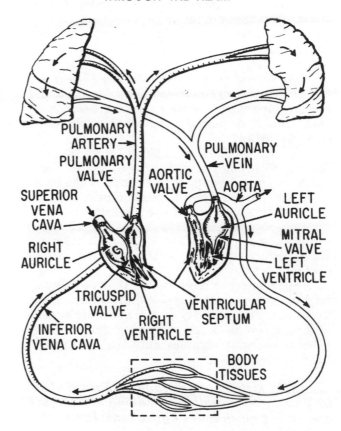

When anemia, thyroid trouble or diabetes are at the root of the trouble, these must be controlled — but that still does not mean that the heart can with impunity be forced beyond its capacity.

Reduction of smoking, or quitting entirely, is wise, because tobacco aggravates angina.

In a few cases of certain types, modern heart surgery can be very useful.

Last, but by no means the least important, emotional stresses and disturbances can evoke pain. Make a conscious effort to avoid getting stirred up. In short, be philosophical about life; it will make you more comfortable.

What is an aneurysm and what causes it? Is there any cure?

An aneurysm is a weak or bulgy spot in a blood vessel. What causes it? Sometimes an injury, but more likely a flaw or weak spot that finally has begun to give way. Arteriosclerosis — arterial hardening — is a common cause.

Aneurysm may occur in any part of the body. In certain areas (such as in the brain) there may be nothing to do about it except to control one's blood pressure, so as to expose the weak spot to as little extra stress as possible.

In still other areas, accessible for surgery, a plastic tube may be inserted to replace the aneurysm.

A dissecting aneurysm is another type. I'll explain. Since an artery consists of an inner and outer layer, if blood seeps through the inner lining the two layers are gradually forced apart. Thus the separation of the layers spreads along the artery, increasing the extent of the aneurysm.

The school doctor has told my 17-year-old son he has a heart murmur. The family and I are very worried. Please explain a heart murmur. Can it be cured, and what precautions must be taken?

A "murmur" is an unusual sound that can be heard through a stethoscope. Some slight variance from average in the shape of the heart or of a valve can cause a small gurgle, whisper or swirling sound out of the ordinary.

A school doctor doesn't have the time to evaluate, much less follow up, such a murmur. He therefore reports it, so the patient's regular doctor can take over.

Some surveys have shown that as many as half or more of all school children have heart murmurs. The majority of murmurs don't mean illness; a few do. Merely knowing that you have a heart murmur signifies only that you should have it checked.

Is the method of determining normal blood pressure still a matter of adding 100 to your age, or is a much lower figure considered satisfactory?

The 100-plus-age "rule" has been bandied about for a long time, but it isn't a very good one. It would be best if we all could keep the same blood pressure we had at the age of 15 or 20, but we can't. As we grow older, our arteries lose their elasticity, and to varying degrees they tend to become somewhat lined with fatty materials.

In consequence, it is that much harder to force the proper blood supply through them. Hence the blood pressure rises. This puts added strain on the heart, as well as other important organs through which the blood flows. The liver, kidneys, lungs, ears, eyes, brain and others may be damaged from too much pressure, too long sustained. Or the blood vessels themselves may rupture.

The formula of 100 plus your age was nothing but guesswork, and the guess was too high. The healthiest people are those whose blood

pressure does NOT rise that fast as they grow older.

Besides, the pumping pressure is not the only important element. The resting pressure (between beats) is very important, too, so our blood pressure is represented as, say, 125/80, the first number being the pumping (or systolic) pressure, and the second being the resting (or diastolic) pressure.

Let's say that one person's reading is 140/95, and another's is 130/110. The second person's systolic pressure is lower — and hence you'd think it would be "better." However, the "resting" pressure is so high that such a reading would make a doctor begin to wonder at once what was wrong, whereas the "higher" pressure of the first patient would cause no alarm.

Can I improve circulation in the legs through exercise?

Yes, but remember that something other than exercise may be a more basic answer. It depends on the cause of the impaired circulation. If, for one instance, varicose veins are the cause, exercise will not take the place of surgical or other treatment.

The so-called Buerger's exercise is simple and excellent when some moderate help to the circulation is necessary, such as massage. Lie on your back. Raise first one leg, then lower it and raise the other. Keep each leg raised for a short time — half a minute, a minute. Raising the leg helps blood flow back toward the heart. Lowering it permits an easy flow of fresh blood.

There's not much to the exercise, but it has proved surprisingly helpful to many people. This we call upside down bicycle riding.

Excessive smoking can impair leg circulation.

I am a middle-aged woman taking, under my physician's direction, quinine sulfate for painful leg cramps which bother me especially in bed at night.

What is the connection between the cramps and poor circulation, which I have been told is the cause? Does this mean my heart is not functioning properly? I seem to be in excellent health otherwise but am exhausted because I can't sleep due to the cramps.

Poor circulation is only one of the causes of leg cramps. If the leg muscles do not get an adequate blood supply, they can go into spasm. These are the cramps.

Such poor circulation does not imply heart disease. Hardening of the arteries can be involved, or there may be some narrowing of the large arteries to the legs at a strategic point, so that interference in circulation is confined to that part of the body, although the heart is operating normally.

Therefore I hope you won't add worry over

your heart to the trouble you already have with the leg cramps. Were your heart involved, your doctor would have noted it already.

What does a C.B.C. mean? My aunt just had one and she has cancer.

C.B.C. means complete blood count. Actually it doesn't mean that every possible blood test is included, because there are all sorts of specialized ones that need be done only when tracking down some particular problem.

Various blood tests, such as, for example, for syphilis, sugar tolerance, or red blood count, or others, might be wanted at times.

The C.B.C. would show a broader spectrum of data, among them anemia, which is often a secondary consequence of cancer. Naturally your aunt's doctor wants to know about this. But a C.B.C. doesn't have any special significance as regards cancer. It applies in all sorts of conditions.

Is there such a thing as a silent heart attack? What are the symptoms, and is the treatment the same as in other heart attacks?

There can be a heart attack with no symptoms of which the patient is aware.

In actual practice when such heart attacks are discovered later (usually by means of an electrocardiogram) careful questioning by the doctor can often elicit a history of some type of discomfort.

This may have been passed off by the patient as indigestion or muscle strain or any of a variety of other explanations. The discomfort may, indeed, have been so mild that the patient disregarded it or actually forgot about it.

Thus these are not really "silent" heart attacks, but have been mistaken for something else.

I wouldn't say that treatment would be the same as in other heart attacks. They simply aren't discovered at the same time, and that makes a lot of difference.

What is pericarditis? How dangerous is it? What causes it and how long is a patient affected by it?

There's a protective sac around the heart called the pericardium. The word comes from "peri," meaning around, and "cardia," meaning heart.

The inner lining of this sometimes becomes inflamed, and that is pericarditis.

COMPOSITION OF THE BLOOD

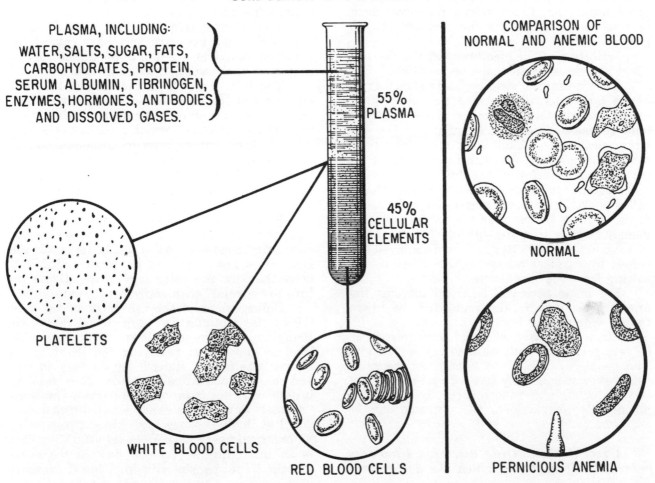

PLASMA, INCLUDING:
WATER, SALTS, SUGAR, FATS, CARBOHYDRATES, PROTEIN, SERUM ALBUMIN, FIBRINOGEN, ENZYMES, HORMONES, ANTIBODIES AND DISSOLVED GASES.

55% PLASMA

45% CELLULAR ELEMENTS

COMPARISON OF NORMAL AND ANEMIC BLOOD

NORMAL

PERNICIOUS ANEMIA

PLATELETS

WHITE BLOOD CELLS

RED BLOOD CELLS

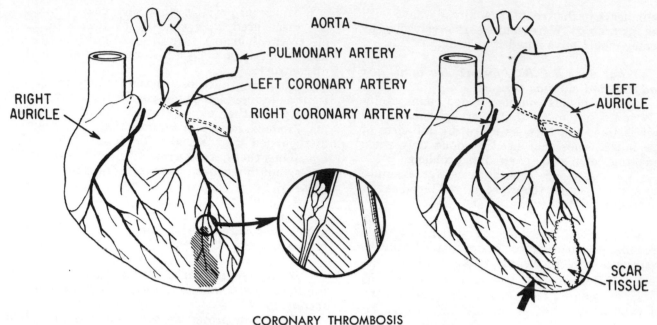

CORONARY THROMBOSIS
Left: At time of attack. Flow of blood through part of the left coronary artery is blocked (insert), cutting off circulation in shade area. Right: Recovery from attack. Scar tissue has built up, blood vessels of right coronary artery (arrow) now supply the affected areas.

Infections are a major cause of pericarditis: Rheumatic fever or other bacterial infections; secondary infections as from pneumonia; virus infections; tuberculosis. Whatever germ is involved, if it inflames the pericardium, it's pericarditis.

Irritation of the membrane at the site of a heart attack can also cause pericarditis.

The rheumatic, viral or heart attack types of irritation usually subside as the original cause is corrected. The other types, however, tend to cause fluid to accumulate in the sac, either clear or pus-filled. Such cases are usually more prolonged and may call for tapping of the pericardium to draw off the fluid.

In some instances scar tissue forms. This is called constrictive pericarditis, since the sac is drawn tighter by the scar tissue, and this, obviously, makes it more difficult for the heart to function. Constrictive pericarditis is usually helped by surgical release of the adhesions resulting from the scar tissue.

For acute pericarditis, the symptoms embrace fever, pain in the region of the heart, cough, shortness of breath.

Since the consequences of pericarditis can be very serious, I don't want to say anything to lead people to take it too lightly. At the same time, when it is quickly treated and the patient is wise enough to follow carefully all of the physician's instructions, the outcome can be excellent.

A recent chest X-ray disclosed I have an enlarged left ventricle which the doctor says was caused by high blood pressure. I am taking medication for the blood pressure. How serious is this condition, and will it cause a heart attack?

Your doctor is quite right when he says that high blood pressure may have caused the enlarged ventricle, but no, it is not the sort of problem which causes a heart attack.

The left ventricle is the last of the four chambers of the heart through which the blood is, in rotation, pumped. When it is called upon to work harder than normal, it tends to enlarge. And working harder usually, although not always, means that something is impeding the blood flow. The heart works harder — and the pressure increases. That's what high blood pressure is all about, really.

Enlargement of the heart, in itself, is not serious. This can result from some severe yet temporary condition. Afterwards, however, the heart does not return to its former size, any more than the muscular legs of an athlete return to "normal" with retirement from sports.

Enlargement of the heart (or of the ventricle) is common in high blood pressure. Bringing the pressure down to a reasonable level is important; restoring the heart to its former size is not. Indeed, hearts vary in size and shape to some degree, as do noses, making it difficult if not impossible to narrow the word "normal" down to an exact set of dimensions.

But don't confuse high blood pressure or an enlarged heart with a "heart attack," which is an interruption of blood flow to the heart muscle. True, people with high blood pressure sometimes have heart attacks, but so do people without it.

I have just returned home after 25 days in the hospital because of a heart attack. Could you explain a machine they kept on me for about four days? I think it is called a heart monitor.

A heart monitor is an instrument essentially similar to an electrocardiograph except that instead of making a tracing on a strip of paper, the tracing appears on a cathode ray screen — the same sort of screen that a TV set has.

Doctors and nurses can see instantly if any change occurs in heart action, instead of having to look at the paper tape.

More and more hospitals have coronary care units that are specifically designed for patients who have had myocardial infarctions.

If a person has low blood presure, does it always stay that way?

It doesn't necessarily remain low. However, there are some people whose blood pressure is naturally low, and it will stay that way. It's nothing for them to be alarmed about in most cases.

Please explain cerebral spasm or ischemia. What causes this?

These are not exactly the same thing.

Ischemia is a lack of sufficient blood supply; the tissues are deprived of necessary nutrients. This can happen in any part of the body — heart, kidneys, brain or elsewhere. The usual cause is clogging or other defect in an artery supplying the area.

If this occurs in the brain, then it is cerebral ischemia.

This occurs only rarely because of spasm, or constriction of an artery, since a spasm is ordinarily brief and so are its effects.

Nicotine can cause such spasms, and this is the reason for the temporary dizziness sometimes experienced by people just beginning to smoke, or by occasional smokers.

The more likely cause of cerebral ischemia is arteriosclerosis, or thickening of the lining of an artery (or arteries); the blood flow is diminished.

If a patient (or his doctor) can detect signs that he may be a likely candidate for a heart attack, can anything be done?

Yes. The danger is that something will occur to shut off the flow of blood through some part of the coronary artery. One of the biggest risks of this sort is that a clot will form, blocking a branch of that vital artery.

An attack, therefore, may be forestalled by the use of anticoagulants, to prevent formation of clots.

We'd best keep in mind that the anticoagulants, useful as they are, won't always work miracles. There are many "ifs" involved. Nor can anticoagulants be used as casually as you might take an aspirin.

Some less dramatic but extremely useful measures may in the long run be more important. One is the matter of overweight. Along with it is the presence of excessive quantities of lipids (fats — including cholesterol) in the blood. Weight reduction, along with limitation of the amount of animal fat in the diet will help.

There was an article in the news about a man who had a physical examination, including a cardiogram, which was said to be perfect; yet a few hours later he died of a heart attack.

People would have a great deal more confidence and trust in the medical profession if they knew the reason for such blunders, or errors, or lack of knowledge.

Perhaps you could clarify this.

It's a shock. It is always hard to believe. It isn't frequent, but it does happen, and it is so dramatically tragic that it gets talked about a great deal.

But it isn't a blunder. It isn't an error. It is lack of knowledge only in the sense that we cannot foretell the future.

An electrocardiogram (EKG or ECG) is a test which, among other things, discloses whether the heart muscle is getting a reasonably adequate supply of blood. If circulation is deficient, the EKG will show an abnormal pattern. If circulation is adequate, the pattern will be normal.

But suppose that the blood supply is shut off? Then you have a heart attack. This may or may not be fatal. The majority of attacks are not.

What causes such a shutting off of circulation? The likeliest cause is the formation of a blood clot which becomes lodged somewhere in the coronary artery or one of its branches. (Some unusual stress, mental or physical, may also perhaps cause a spasm or narrowing which may lead to clogging.)

This we cannot predict. There are too many variables. Such an accident, from whatever combination of events, can (and does) sometimes occur immediately after a test has shown adequate blood supply. There is no error, no blunder. But we don't have a crystal ball.

I have been advised by my doctor to have a pacemaker implanted for my slow-beating heart. I am now taking medication every four hours around the clock, but the doctor said he wanted to see me in six months, which means I may have to have the heart surgery then. What do you think about such an operation?

A "slow heart" or fast or irregular heart

can be speeded up to some extent by medicines, but they have to be taken constantly. A pacemaker has two main advantages. One is that it requires very little attention and you can sleep through the night without medication. The other is that the rate of heart beat can be set at the speed which best suits your needs, whereas medication cannot always achieve optimum rate.

The pacemaker is a miniaturized instrument which releases small electric impulses. You do not feel them, but they are strong enough to cause the heart muscle to contract.

An electrode leading from the pacemaker is embedded in the heart muscle itself. The pacemaker is placed inside the chest, close below the surface.

The operation, compared to others which are being performed every day, is rather simple. In the heart itself, all that is necessary is placement of the electrode.

The reason for putting the pacemaker inside the body instead of outside is that, if a wire is run through the skin, festering may begin at the point of entry.

The pacemaker uses but little current and modern miniature batteries are so efficient that they will last for several years before requiring replacement. Even then, it is quite simple. The whole operation doesn't have to be repeated. It is necessary only to open the surface tissues enough to gain access to the battery.

What about the drug digitalis, its merits and also its dangers?

Digitalis is an old drug but it remains one of the most important. It was introduced into medicine 185 years ago by an English physician, Withering, and we have yet to find anything that is as good as this for necessary uses.

The drug is obtained from the dried leaves of the foxglove, a common garden flower. Strangely enough, chemists still have not been able to make it synthetically.

Digitalis strengthens the beat of a weakened heart muscle. A weak heart beats rapidly but with little force.

With the use of digitalis, the heart rate becomes slower, the force of each beat is substantially increased, and total circulation is augmented. It is wonderfully effective.

In some patients with irregular heart rhythm, such as auricular fibrillation, digitalis is effective in stabilizing the rhythm. The drug has no effect on a normal heart.

Dosage is gauged by the patient's need and his response. Once the maintenance dose — the amount required to keep the heart operating well — is established, that amount should be taken daily because the effect is lost if the drug is stopped or even omitted for a short time. A valuable but curious medicine, isn't it?

The dangers? They are few. Overdosage can slow the heart rate excessively. Overdosage also can cause nausea, vomiting and diarrhea. In some individuals, but this is rare, it can cause yellow vision — everything they look at seems to have a yellowish cast.

I read your article on digitalis and would like one on nitroglycerin.

Nitroglycerin is possibly the most useful drug we have for one type of heart trouble, angina pectoris, which is chest pain resulting (usually) from insufficient blood circulation to the heart muscle.

After exertion, or a big meal which is an activity that puts demands on blood circulation, the heart muscle, overtaxed, cramps painfully.

Resting the heart until it catches up its strength, is important. But a tiny amount of nitroglycerin, acting as a drug, does it quicker. It dilates the coronary arteries, allowing more blood to flow, but without increasing the work of the heart. Other drugs will improve circulation, but they also put added strain on the heart.

That is why nitroglycerin is so useful. There is a similar preparation, amyl nitrite, which also is very effective but its effects are not as long-lasting. A tablet of nitroglycerin brings relief within minutes, and the effects last from 30 minutes to several hours, depending on the patient. (The tablets are dissolved under the tongue, which is much more effective than swallowing them.)

There can be some side effects which the patient should be warned about: A feeling of fullness in the head, transient giddiness, flushing or warmth of the skin. Once one gets used to them — if they occur — they are usually well tolerated, and certainly preferable to the exhausting pain of an attack.

Here's another warning: Nitroglycerin must be used cautiously by patients with glaucoma; if you have glaucoma, make sure your doctor is told about it.

Nitroglycerin is inexpensive, and not habit-forming.

Please explain tachycardia. What are its symptoms and causes? How can you avoid it? Is it dangerous?

Tachycardia simply means rapid heart beat. When it occurs because of fright, excitement or violent exercise, we are not concerned. (Fever, shock and excessive bleeding are other causes.)

But when we detect no reason for it, then we become worried, naturally.

Yet again, an overactive thyroid can cause it. This can be a very subtle thing in older persons, and baffling until identified.

But in the overall picture, keep in mind that the "pacemaker" which controls the heart rate is by and large very orderly. When it does depart from its normal rate, it can affect either the upper chambers of the heart (auricles) or the lower chambers (ventricles).

In the former case, heart disease usually is NOT present, especially if the rhythm, while speeded up, is regular. However, irregular beating, or fibrillation, requires additional examination.

With rapid beating of the ventricles, there is likelihood of some form of heart disease. The patient doesn't know whether the upper or lower chambers are involved, but the doctor does and this gives him an immediate clue.

Symptoms of tachycardia? A sense of palpitation of the heart, light-headedness sometimes, shortness of breath, a "gassy" feeling. If overactive thyroid is involved, the speeded-up heart beat can be continuous. With the usually harmless speed-up of the auricles, it can start suddenly, last for an indefinite time, from a few minutes to several hours or even days, and then stop as abruptly as it began.

I understand that bicycle riding is excellent exercise for heart patients. I ride every day and, as I have angina, I wonder if you approve. I don't notice any bad effects.

I approve, subject to several qualifications. Under normal circumstances bicycle riding is mild, pleasant exercise.

Dr. Paul Dudley White popularized it. However, many other forms of exercise are just as good: not excessively strenuous, but steady and pleasant. But some may not suit your temperament and circumstances, or lend themselves as well to daily use. It may not be as easy (or it may, for some, be easier!) to do a little swimming, a little bowling, some calisthenics, a little work in the garden, some walking, some work in a basement workshop, paddling a canoe or rowing a boat. Golf, leisurely, probably 9 holes rather than 18, on a not-too-hilly course, is also acceptable.

All of us need exercise unless some problem of health interferes.

For the person with angina, if bicycle riding causes no bad effects — either shortness of breath or pain — it is good exercise. Any form of steady and regular exercise within those limitations is good. It will strengthen the heart by gradually increasing circulation through development of small blood vessels. Overdoing, indicated by pain or breathlessness, will not help. It will do damage.

Relative to blood transfusions, there is a belief by some people that the patient acquires some characteristics of the donor.

If so, is it possible for a criminal donor to pass on his tendencies? Please explain how blood tends to fuse into the body and brain of the patient receiving it.

This is not true. First of all, the permanent characteristics of a person are determined by the chromosomes, and the thousands or perhaps millions of genes contained in the original cell, half from the mother, half from the father.

True, the developing fetus may be damaged (as in birth defects) but this is DAMAGE, and not a change in fundamentals. Color of hair and eyes, shape of face and body, inherited strengths and weaknesses, are controlled by genes — not in any way by blood.

It has been customary to speak of "blood lines," a term which was used long before we had the faintest idea of what the genes are and how they behave, but that old expression still gives rise to a lot of false beliefs.

Blood — the fluid, and the cells in it — serves principally as a "delivery service," carrying oxygen, sugar and other nutrients throughout the body, and carrying away debris and waste matter. The blood carries oxygen from the lungs; it carries carbon dioxide back to the lungs to be exhaled. It also carries antibodies to fight off infections. But it does not control our characteristics.

When you have a need for blood and require a transfusion, you don't keep that blood permanently. In a matter of three months or less, all of the transfused blood cells will have died off and been discarded by the body.

Gradually new cells will have replaced the old ones, and the new ones will be your own, created in the marrow of your bones.

Phrases about "blood lines," or "a taint in the blood" should be abolished from the language, because blood has nothing to do with the kind of people we are.

What about the blood disease known as mononucleosis? Is it spread only by saliva? Can it recur, or may one have it once and become immune?

It seems to be spreading among teenagers.

Infectious mononucleosis is a virus infection. It is characterized (and thus named) by the presence in the blood of a large number of white cells, called mononuclear ones. A blood test is an excellent way of diagnosing a suspected case, but this does not imply that treatment of the blood is necessary.

Rather, mononucleosis is a self-limiting disease. Like the common cold, you get it and you get over it, and there isn't any specific cure.

Whether it is spread "only by saliva" is not known, but it does spread from person to person, especially among young people, and often among college students in dormitories or troops in military installations.

The characteristics include fatigue, swollen and tender glands (it is also called "glandular fever"), and sometimes a transient hepatitis — that is, a liver condition, but not to be confused with the more serious types.

Plenty of rest and wholesome food, and

precautions against complications, are the essential treatment. Taking the ailment too lightly isn't wise, because relapses can occur.

On the other hand, it isn't the type of ailment that should frighten anyone. It clears up, leaving no after-effects. One attack usually confers immunity, which very possibly may be why we see it among young people and rarely among older ones.

I question whether it really is "spreading among teenagers," but suspect, rather, that it is being diagnosed more readily instead of being passed off as something else.

Exactly how the virus is transmitted is not known. Mononucleosis has been called "the kissing disease" because of the age of its most frequent victims, but that doesn't explain its spread in non-coeducational schools or army barracks. It may spread pretty much the way colds do, or measles, or whatnot.

What can be done for pernicious anemia? I have had it for years. I take medication and eat liver several times a week. Has a cure been found for it?

No cure has been found, but it can be readily kept under control by periodic injections of Vitamin B_{12}. Liver is high in this vitamin. Before the important ingredient was narrowed down to B_{12}, it was necessary for patients to eat liver daily and in extremely large quantities.

I went to donate blood and the bank wouldn't take it. They told me I was anemic and to go home and take a tonic. What causes this and what should I do about it?

I hope the next anemic person who visits a blood bank will be advised to see his doctor.

Anemia means either that the normal number of red blood cells are not present or a deficiency in iron exists.

There are many kinds of anemia, and just as many causes, and no single form of treatment or "tonic" will fit all of them. You can't get anywhere by guesswork. But with certain blood tests your doctor can readily tell a great deal about which type of anemia is present, and what to do about it.

One is just from loss of blood — a bleeding ulcer, hemorrhoids, excessive menstruation. Sometimes the patient does not even know it.

Anyway, red cells may be lost faster than the body can provide new ones. The result? Anemia.

Or faulty nutrition may be and often is the cause. The red cells contain hemoglobin (to carry fresh oxygen) and iron is vital for the creation of hemoglobin. So iron may be given in one form or another. (That's the "tonic" mentioned to you.)

Yet there may be iron enough, but a lack of something else: Adequate protein, or tiny traces of copper which are necessary chemically if the body is to use iron properly, and probably Vitamin C and other vitamins must be present.

In still other cases, a blood disorder may cause the red cells to be of the wrong size or shape, and thus unable to carry out their assigned duties. And there is pernicious anemia, once a very dangerous disease indeed, but now controlled readily by periodic injections of Vitamin B_{12}.

There are other and more complicated forms of anemia, but they are rare.

By and large, most of the anemias can be very effectively treated, once the particular type has been determined.

INHERITANCE OF THE BLOOD GROUPS

Blood Groups of Parents	Blood Groups which may occur in Children	Blood Groups which do not occur in Children
O × O	O	A, B, AB
O × A	O, A	B, AB
A × A	O, A	B, AB
O × B	O, B	A, AB
B × B	O, B	A, AB
A × B	O, A, B, AB	—
O × AB	A, B	O, AB
A × AB	A, B, AB	O
B × AB	A, B, AB	O
AB × AB	A, B, AB	O

Copyright 1951 Laurence H. Snyder and D. C. Heath and Co.

I understand that leukemia is a very deadly disease, but my father, now in his 60's, has had it for some years and still goes to work every day.

The fundamental characteristic of leukemia is the production of too many white cells in the blood, at the expense of other necessary elements. (White cells are invaluable in protection against disease, but occasionally they develop in excessive numbers, and in immature, useless form.)

You must keep this in mind: There are two major types, acute leukemia, which primarily affects children, and the chronic, slow-developing form, more frequent in adults.

Children, if they developed leukemia, used to die within a matter of months. Today it is still an ominous disease, but with steroids, transfusions and special drugs, life may be prolonged in some cases for five years or so. In some exceptional cases, a few have survived for upwards of 10. But we cannot say that a "cure" is yet possible.

The chronic cases in older adults are quite different. With adequate treatment, the older patient with chronic leukemia looks good, feels good, pursues his usual occupation, may go on comfortably for 20 years. Such a patient requires constant vigilance by his doctor, and appropriate treatment when it is needed.

Skin Disorders, Allergies & Asthma

COMBINING THESE seemingly varied disorders into a single chapter is somewhat arbitrary but not without a reason.

The skin is the largest organ of the body. It includes the hair and nails, and it is well to remember that hair and nail ailments are part of the specialty of the dermatologist or skin specialist.

A myriad of troubles can afflict the skin, and while some types are easy enough to describe, others are not. Except to an expert, some skin ailments look so much like wholly different ones that the patient may jump to a wrong conclusion.

With transient, unimportant skin ailments, this may not make much difference. But there are too many times when a person decides that he has "eczema," and tries to doctor himself with a variety of salves or other remedies.

Dermatologists complain that by the time they see a case, sometimes the remedies have actually done enough irritating (in addition to scratching or other injury to the skin) that bacterial infection has been added on top of the original condition and it becomes difficult to determine what the original trouble was, and treatment is difficult.

Allergies, or contact dermatitis, are a large factor in skin eruptions of various types. Most folks will get a rash from poison ivy, if they are sufficiently exposed to it — but some are much more sensitive than others.

Still other individuals, however, will be hyper-sensitive, or allergic, to materials which are totally harmless to others. Some are sensitive to metals, even good jewelry. Nickel- or chrome-plated scissors may make one's fingers break out. Metal desk tops, carbon paper, hair dyes, shaving lotions, medicated soaps, all sorts of cosmetics, dust, flowers, fabrics — some people have been troubled by all of these. The list is endless.

Thus it is impossible to discuss skin disorders without considering allergies. But allergies can cause troubles other than skin rashes, itching, or hives. They can inflame nose and eyes (hay fever, etc.). They can cause sneezing — one man had a violent attack whenever a bartender peeled a lemon, some feet away from him.

Allergies can interfere with digestion, cause the lips to swell, touch off certain types of headaches, cause swelling of tissues in the respiratory system.

That last aspect becomes important because of the vast number of asthma cases which exist. While in adults, other circumstances may contribute to asthma (the cardiac asthma of a heart patient, for one), in children allergy should be the first suspicion when asthma develops.

I always used to have nice fingernails, but they have become very weak, break and split easily, and I just cannot keep them looking nice. I have heard that taking plain gelatin every day will harden them.

Gelatin, so highly publicized for the nails, simply is not a specific for hardening them. Only by coincidence is it likely to help. There are several known reasons for brittle nails.

1. Faulty diet, particularly deficiency of protein and/or calcium, is one. True, gelatin is protein, but it is an "incomplete protein," containing only some of the amino acids. Be sure you get ample protein in the form of lean meat, eggs, fish, cheese. A couple of glasses of milk a day (skim milk or low-fat if you prefer) will assure calcium.

2. General health is highly important. A

checkup including tests for anemia or low thyroid, is wise. Faulty circulation also can be a factor.

3. Some nail polishes or removers may bother a few individuals.

4. Nails, like other tissues, become stronger from use. People who do hard manual labor seldom have weak nails. It is feminine fashion to want long, carefully shaped nails. Result: Women naturally try to protect the nails by putting as little pressure on them as possible. The nails thus lose instead of gain strength. And, of course, the length of the nails makes breakage more likely.

My niece wants me to go to a specialist with her to have her freckles removed. She said there is a method called sandpaper surgery that removes freckles. Just what is this, and what is the approximate cost? Is it dangerous?

Skin-planing or dermabrasion is a better term than sandpaper surgery, and it is done by plastic surgeons and some dermatologists. It consists of removing the outer layer of skin, usually with a high speed revolving drum, with an abrasive surface. This has to be done under completely sterile conditions. Then a new layer of skin replaces that which has been removed.

Since the skin actually is removed, the freckles will go with it — but what's to prevent new freckles from forming? If your niece hasn't thought of this, she should. The procedure is not cheap — and not guaranteed.

My 3-year-old daughter has had eczema since she was 7 months old. Doctors prescribed a lotion to use several times a day, but she still has the disease. It is on her arms and neck, and sometimes on her ears.

Should I have her take tests to see whether there's a food allergy?

Eczema, like some other ailments, is a general term that can mean different things. It is a skin disorder — but the problem is to pinpoint the cause.

Except for transient skin irritations, a lotion isn't the answer, although it naturally helps to relieve itching while a diagnosis is being sought.

Frequently a food allergy is the cause of eczema in children, so your suggestion of tests is good. Egg white, cow's milk and various grains such as wheat, barley, corn and oats are among the most frequent offenders.

However, a contact allergy may be involved — a reaction to something she touches. The fact that the trouble is confined mostly to her arms and neck could be a clue in this direction.

Wool, silk, or other fabrics are known to trigger such a skin sensitivity, as can something in the fabrics, such as dye or sizing or whatever. Skin tests may give a definite clue as to either type of allergy — food or contact. Consult an allergist.

What can I do to get rid of dandruff? I have tried all sorts of shampoos but my scalp still becomes itchy and it scales when I scratch.

Dandruff is a fairly common problem. Let's examine what dandruff really is. It is a flaking of the outer layers of skin in the scalp. That's what those white specks are — skin, in tiny particles.

The cause won't be the same in all cases, so neither will the remedy. Usually, dandruff is associated with excessive secretion of oil glands in the scalp. A scaliness results and it in turn produces itching. So you scratch. And the skin flakes.

As a rule one of the readily available shampoos takes care of the condition. However, keep this in mind: With a good deal of scratching, the skin can have become broken, allowing little infections to start — sometimes bacteria, sometimes fungus. And that, naturally, makes the whole condition worse.

What can be done for cold sores? I frequently break out with four or five of them on my lip. Some people believe this to be hereditary and others think it is a nervous condition.

Neither heredity nor nerves is the cause. It's a virus (Herpes simplex). There is considerable medical opinion to the effect that some people are exposed to it in childhood but do not acquire any immunity to it as they do to other germs. The virus remains (according to this belief, which is plausible) and breaks out into a new cold sore when resistance lags, as when you have a cold, get too tired, etc. A smallpox vaccination stops the trouble for some people. For others, it doesn't, and the application of a drying agent, as a camphor lotion, is about all that you can do.

I have children, aged one and two. My daughter had impetigo when she was five months old, and now my son has it. I keep them as clean as I can. What can I do to get rid of this condition?

Impetigo is an infection of the skin, not only infectious (caused by germs) but contagious (passed from person to person).

True, cleanliness is extremely important but that isn't the whole story. Despite all reasonable care, it is still possible for the infection to spread because you can't see the germs. They may be transmitted by a child touching another, or by use of another's handkerchief, toys, pencils or whatnot.

In this case there is at least a hint that the disease may have been passed, not from child to child, but from adult to child.

Someone in or close to the household may be a carrier of the germs, more particularly the staphylococcus variety. This has been known to happen many times and is one of the threats against which well-run nurseries are constantly on guard.

These germs can be carried in the nose, cause no trouble to the carrier, yet become devilishly mean if they reach a person who possesses poor protection against them.

It sometimes is necessary to have laboratory cultures grown and examined from nose and throat swabbings of others in the family, especially the parents, and I think that is the logical starting point in this case.

Is shingles a virus that attacks the nerves, or is it due to nervousness? If it is a virus, then can't it be transmitted?

A member of our family has awful dark splotches all over her skin and apparently it itches very much. We were told it is shingles, but she is not taking any medication for it, nor has she had a doctor. We are very concerned as there are several small children in the family.

Yes, shingles is a virus infection of a nerve trunk, and it is NOT nervousness. Yes, shingles can be transmitted.

Shingles is an ailment of the middle-aged and older. Its counterpart in children is chicken pox. The viruses of the two diseases are very similar.

How the relative with the splotchy itch can know what this trouble is, without having medical advice, I can't say. She may have some sort of skin disease which, unless treated, may be worse than shingles, and for all I know may be more dangerous for the children.

My suggestion is to tell her that somebody said it is "Herpes zoster," and she should see her doctor. I leave it to your discretion whether to tell her that "Herpes zoster" is merely the technical term for shingles.

What causes athlete's foot and what makes it come and go? Is there any cure for it? What will stop the itching? Is it a skin disease?

Yes, it's a skin disease. A fungus becomes attached to the skin and begins to grow. Think of it like mold that grows on a piece of bread, except that the fungus is much smaller.

Let's suppose that you get rid of almost all of the fungus, and your feet seem to be cured. But a little of the fungus remains. It starts to spread, and finally reaches a stage at which you notice it again. That's the principal explanation of why the disease seems to come and go.

Yes, you can cure athlete's foot, but one thing you must keep in mind: Treatment should continue after you think you have it beaten. Why? Because if a little trace of the fungus

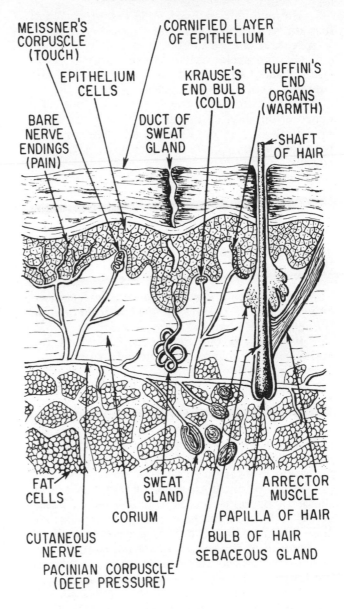

MEISSNER'S CORPUSCLE (TOUCH)
EPITHELIUM CELLS
BARE NERVE ENDINGS (PAIN)
CORNIFIED LAYER OF EPITHELIUM
KRAUSE'S END BULB (COLD)
DUCT OF SWEAT GLAND
RUFFINI'S END ORGANS (WARMTH)
SHAFT OF HAIR
FAT CELLS
CUTANEOUS NERVE
PACINIAN CORPUSCLE (DEEP PRESSURE)
SWEAT GLAND
CORIUM
ARRECTOR MUSCLE
PAPILLA OF HAIR
BULB OF HAIR
SEBACEOUS GLAND

remains, it can start to grow again. Since the fungus gets itself rooted right in the skin, and can hide in layers of dead skin, or in or under the nails, you have to keep at the treatment after you seem to have won.

Soaking the feet in a solution of potassium permanganate (1/5,000 dilution) is an old remedy, but an effective one. True, it stains the skin or anything else, and it is toxic if taken internally, so it should be used with care.

A variety of powders, salves and lotions are available, and work — provided you follow directions and don't stop treatment too soon.

Preparations containing griseofulvin, taken by mouth, can be used, but you must remember that not all fungi are the same, and this drug does not combat all of them. In severe, constantly-recurring cases, have your doctor supervise the treatment.

Your own responsibility, whether you are

trying to do it yourself or have your doctor's help, includes these items:

Meticulous foot hygiene is essential. Wash feet daily. Certain skins are more susceptible to infection than others.

Change socks daily, or even oftener. Iron clean socks, since heat and dryness kill the fungus. Wool socks are better than nylon.

Wear different shoes — the same pair only every other day, or better yet only every third or fourth day if possible, to let them dry out between wearings, thus destroying traces of fungus in the shoes.

Dust feet and shoes with foot powder. Modern sprays are excellent, too. Never walk on carpet in bare feet. You may leave the fungus there, and pick it up again later.

Trim and clean toenails as you would fingernails. This gets rid of lurking colonies of the fungus.

My son has a severe case of psoriasis and believes that a no-protein diet will help him. What is your opinion?

Psoriasis is one of the most aggravating maladies we know because nobody to date has found any sure cure for it.

Fortunately psoriasis ordinarily does no harm except to one's appearance, and it is not contagious. It just looks bad!

Different kinds of diet have been tried but have not been found effective. One school believes a high-fat diet is helpful. Another school prefers a low-fat, high protein routine.

More recently taurine, one of the amino acids, (a protein) has been suspected of being poorly tolerated by psoriasis patients. To reduce intake of taurine, it is necessary to limit the amount of protein from animal sources, and to use special cooking procedures to leach out the taurine.

This is not a "no-protein" diet, but one that restricts it. Care must be exercised in using the diet, especially among adolescents who, still growing, are urgently in need of protein.

Thus any attempt at such a diet should be under strict supervision of your physician.

I don't condemn any sincere and careful method of treating — or trying to treat — psoriasis. In any event, most of the many proposed remedies have seemed to work in certain cases, although since psoriasis can come and go without any visible reason or even stop without any treatment at all, it is hard to say whether a remedy really has worked or just happened to be in use when the psoriasis subsided spontaneously.

Please discuss lack of pigmentation in the skin. My skin is getting worse and seemingly there is nothing that can be done. Is it from lack of vitamins? Is it hereditary?

This is called vitiligo — loss of pigment in patches of skin. Heredity probably is a factor. Certain skin infections can be involved. Damage to the skin (as from severe sunburn) sometimes can leave areas where pigment will not accumulate sufficiently. And other times no specific cause can be detected. I hope it will make you feel better to know that:

1. There is nothing harmful to health in this condition.

2. Sometimes it clears up by itself.

In the interim, cosmetics are probably the most satisfactory answer. Drugs have been tried but without dependable success.

Can a sunlamp to acquire a tan harm the skin? Some people tell me its use might develop into skin cancer.

People who for years are exposed to intense sun are more likely to develop skin cancer. A sunlamp, since it gives off similar ultraviolet rays, could contribute to skin cancer, too. But not quickly, and not from moderate exposure.

Be careful not to get a burn (either from the sun or the lamp). Be satisfied with a gradual and moderate tan. Don't try to make yourself the color of shoe leather. With those precautions, you need have no worry.

What causes hair to turn gray? Mine was always very dark and I assumed that when it began to turn, it would be very white. Instead it has a yellowish tinge. Several beauticians tell me this is caused by an acid condition. How can it be remedied?

Except for treating severe malnutrition, thyroid deficiency and various skin diseases attacking the scalp, there isn't much we can do about controlling the amount, quality and natural color of the hair.

Diseases with high fever sometimes cause loss of hair, but all we can do is treat the disease and hope the hair regrows, which it usually does.

Other than that, heredity appears to be the most important governing factor. The original color is due to pigments. As a person grows older, the amount of pigment declines, principally because of diminished blood supply to the hair follicles, or to enzyme changes which govern the conversion of nutrients into pigments.

In general, these are natural processes. When a person becomes gray very early, it is more likely due to some hereditary defect in the chemistry of pigment formation. People in the best of health become prematurely gray because of this.

Whether the hair then is white or yellowish, depends on the original color, because there can be a mixture of pigments, yellow among others. Darker pigments cover up the yellow; as they fade, the yellow tinge becomes visible.

It is NOT caused by "an acid condition," and beauticians would do their clients a favor by discarding that old wheeze. In fact, acid condition has been used as an explanation for everything from hiccups to hangnails, and used so often that people take it for granted that it means something. Well, it doesn't.

What causes erysipelas? Does it have any connection with the nerves? Is it contagious?

It is caused by one strain of the streptococcus germ infecting the skin and underlying tissues, so the surface appears shiny and swollen, pink or red, and tender.

It is not nearly as common as it used to be, thanks to the antibiotic drugs, but it most frequently attacks people already weakened by some other health problem. If the patient does not throw it off (with the help of medication) it can lead to general infection, kidney disease, pneumonia.

Erysipelas also has a tendency to recur, but it is not particularly contagious, except to women at the time of childbirth.

I am a 15-year-old girl and my hair is about down to the middle of my back. I would like it to be longer but it seems to have stopped growing. Is it true that hair stops at a certain length for each individual?

That is essentially correct. At about 10 inches, the rate of growth declines about 50 per cent. However, there are great variations from person to person. The fastest rate of growth in women is between the ages of 15 and 25, so yours in all probability will grow still longer if you let it.

Is it safe to pinch blackheads and pimples on the face? I have heard both pro and con, even from doctors. Someone else said blackheads, yes, pimples, no.

I have dark, oily skin and get many "white" blackheads. It seems silly to run to a dermatologist for something like this, but I don't want to do anything dangerous to myself, either.

Unfortunately too many people pinch blackheads as though they were trying to crack a walnut or something. Skin can be easily injured — and skin injuries make it easy for infections to start.

Hence people who pinch blackheads often have pimples (a small infection) or infected skin glands following the procedure.

The important thing is to remove blackheads gently. Use a comedone remover (comedone being a technical word for blackhead). This inexpensive little gadget will help you press the blackheads out gently without pinching the skin and tearing the tissues.

Generally speaking it's best not to stir up pimples. A pimple (as opposed to a blackhead or whitehead) indicates that an area of infection has developed but the body's defenses are bringing it under control. (Otherwise it would be inflamed.) So leave it alone and Nature will get rid of it.

Can poison ivy be prevented? What is the best treatment? Why are some people immune?

Nobody is immune, but some people are much less sensitive than others. Sometimes a person experiences only mild discomfort — until finally he becomes sensitized. Then he has trouble, too.

Only sure preventive is to avoid getting the sticky sap of leaves or stem on the skin. Immediate washing with strong soap and a thorough lather can help, however.

If you get the rash, lotions containing zirconium or calomine are soothing. In severe cases, with the skin becoming fiery red, compresses of Burow's solution help. In still more severe cases, a physician can prescribe sprays containing steroids, or give steroids by mouth.

Prevention of ivy poisoning has not been too successful. Injections mostly have proved a disappointment; giving very tiny amounts by mouth, and gradually increasing the dose, can build limited protection for sensitive patients, but they still must try to avoid contact.

While the ivy poison cannot "fly through the air," it can be carried by dust or smoke, or picked up on a dog's fur or on shoes or clothing of others, and thus "mysteriously" transferred to ivy-sensitive people.

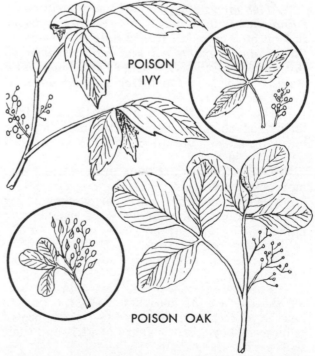

Poison ivy's common east of the Rockies. It has three leaflets, with grayish berries in season. Poison oak is common on West Coast, three leaflets, white berries.

What causes moles and how can one get rid of them? I have them on my neck and now have one in my hair which is getting bigger.

Moles aren't "caused by anything," in the ordinary sense of the words. They aren't there because of anything we do or don't do. They're just there.

Except that they may not look good, moles usually do no harm, so unless you want them removed for the sake of appearance, or unless they show some sign of becoming dangerous, you may leave them alone.

There's nothing you can do yourself about them. They won't bleach, and there is no safe way for you to remove them. However, your doctor can remove them safely.

Incidentally the flat type of mole should be called a nevus. It may be brown or some other color. A strawberry or port wine birthmark is usually a nevus.

A mole, strictly speaking, is both colored and raised. It may or may not have hair. Never pluck hairs from a mole. If they bother you, clip them off with scissors.

The danger signs for moles (or nevi) are these: If they are subject to constant irritation (under a brassiere, strap, belt, or where the razor nicks them while shaving) or if they change size, shape or color, or show any tendency to bleed, they usually should be removed. One risk is cancer. Infection is another.

Thus the one in your hair, since it is changing in size, probably should be removed. Consult a dermatologist.

After much expense and many treatments I find that hair removed by electrolysis seems to be growing back. I would hate to have to do this again. Previously I had hair removed by the hot wax method in a beauty shop and found it satisfactory. Is the latter method harmful to the skin?

The wax method is not particularly irritating, as chemical depilatories may be. The hairs are pulled out, but as you now know, they will grow in again.

Electrolysis is a tedious process and hence more expensive, but it is the only method I know which destroys hair permanently. Any apparent regrowth actually is of neighboring hairs which you may not have noticed, or the follicle was not destroyed by the treatment.

Here's an explanation of the principal methods:

1. Shaving, of course, just cuts the hair off the surface. It does not make the growth heavier or coarser, despite the fond hopes of adolescent boys, or the fears of girls and their mothers.

2. Abrasion used to be popular and effective to the same degree as shaving. Pumice stone rubbed across the skin grinds off the hair.

3. Depilatories are chemicals in cream or other form which dissolve the hair.

4. Wax removal pulls out the hair. The follicles remain, however, and new hair will grow. This is the equivalent of plucking.

5. Electrolysis destroys the follicle, so hair cannot again grow from it — but this does not prevent other follicles from continuing to produce hair. That, in fact, is the basic difficulty with electrolysis. You have to go at it one hair at a time.

I have heard that wearing the hair in a pony tail often can cause baldness. Is this true?

A tight pony tail puts pressure on the roots, and some studies have disclosed that this damages them at times. If you don't pull the tail too tight I doubt if harm will result.

I had naturally curly hair until the births of my two children. Then it straightened out completely. What causes this? I've waited two years, hoping that time and my beautician would restore the curl.

Pregnancy (and anesthesia associated with it) can cause hair loss or change in curl, but the reasons are not apparent. Unfortunately I cannot say whether or not time and your beautician will win out.

I am a woman of 40 and have a problem of hair loss. A physical checkup shows my condition to be normal. In view of this what are the possibilities of hair transplanting?

Transplanting of hair has been done successfully, but it is a fairly new technique. It is painstaking and expensive. Obviously it is also dependent on having enough hair on some areas for transplanting.

For those reasons I am not disposed to recommend that people try it without carefully balancing all the factors.

There is one further and very important thing for you to do. Have a dermatologist examine your scalp. For example, if there is some skin ailment or infection which is causing hair loss, such loss can continue despite the effort and cost of transplanting.

There are different reasons for loss of hair. It is not unusual for women to notice some thinning as they reach 40. Or the loss may be a matter of the hair being brittle and breaking off rather than inability of the follicles to grow hair.

Has your thyroid been checked? Low thyroid activity can be an important factor, and a correctible one.

In some instances the use of certain dyes or other materials applied to the hair may be harmful. Here again a dermatologist can help trace down and identify the trouble.

Nervous problems sometimes produce patchy loss of hair, and correction of them brings regrowth, but this takes time.

Finally, heredity is a strong force which we cannot change. Although baldness is many times more frequent in men than in women, a fair number of women are affected.

Appealing as the idea of transplanting hair is, it isn't an easy solution to the problem. A skilled and deliberate investigation of the type of hair loss is the sensible first step before leaping to the conclusion that transplanting is going to be the answer. I have no doubt that the people who developed the transplanting technique will tell you the same thing.

My 12-year-old daughter has acne. We have tried all kinds of creams and soaps but none has done any good. Do you have any suggestions?

Acne is a frequent plague to youngsters, and if the trouble is going to come, it usually starts on the verge of the teens.

I'm glad you are concerned about it now instead of later. The sooner you start combatting the trouble, the less total damage will be done.

Acne is a consequence of the process of growing up. The body's glandular system becomes more active, and this includes the tiny sebaceous glands of the skin.

These glands normally produce sebum, an oily material which lubricates the skin. If it is produced too rapidly, it clogs outlets of the glands, and the glands then swell into the red blemishes of acne.

These are unsightly, but the worst consequence is that some of them become pustules — infected spots. This is what does the serious scarring and pitting of the skin.

How do you avoid this? First, the pores must be kept open, so the oily sebum will have less chance to clog. Scrupulous hygiene is mandatory. Nothing will take its place. Washing several times a day is a chore, but it is worth the trouble. And the rinsing is extremely important. Use a great deal of fresh, warm or tepid water to rinse away everything that the washing has loosened up.

Use of creams and special soaps can be disappointing unless you know exactly what you are trying to accomplish. Some creams, in fact, may aggravate the condition.

Diet also must be considered — a reduction in fats and sugars. There is some evidence that reduction in milk intake may be beneficial since it contains fats and sugars. Use of chocolate and other confections relished by growing youngsters may have to be curtailed. Emotional disturbances are also a factor.

It is well worthwhile to have your doctor's help when battling acne.

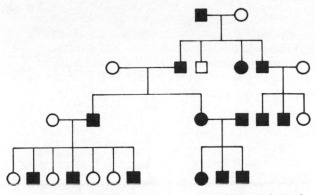

This pedigree of baldness in a family indicates how the characteristic was passed along by great grandfather to 3 of his children, 5 grandchildren, and 6 great grandchildren. Twelve of the 15 bald persons were males. (Square symbols are males; bald persons are in black.)

For four years my son has been going to a dermatologist for an acne condition.

All kinds of salves and medications have been used but the most beneficial treatment has been 50,000 units of Vitamin A a day. How long is it safe to give this much?

Vitamin A, in some (but not all) cases seems to be helpful. We don't know why. However, some dermatologists think it is useless.

It should not be used (at the rate of 50,000 units a day) for more than six months running. At such a rate, for that long, it can become toxic with such symptoms as hair loss, weakness, loss of appetite, yellowish color of the palms.

If it seems to help, use it for two or three months, then stop use of it for a month to prevent such unwanted symptoms.

What about food allergies? My 13-year-old daughter has sniffles and sneezes and to ascertain the cause the doctor made tests which showed she has a tendency to be allergic to the following: Milk (she loves it), corn oil, beef, eggs and chicken.

Allergy or atopy (allergy to foods) is one of the commonest of ailments — a hypersensitivity.

It can be sensitivity to something you breathe (hay fever), or touch (contact dermatitis, detergent hands, etc.), something you eat, or even such things as sun, cold, etc.

The best solution is to avoid whatever allergen affects you, if possible. This applies to foods as well as other factors.

Allergic reactions have a tendency to add up. You may be able to stand a little of something, but a lot of it touches off the allergy. Or you may be allergic to a number of things. If you encounter several of them at the same time, trouble may result even though, singly, the same things do not offend.

Eggs and milk are rather frequent foods involving allergy. While milk is valuable, if it proves to bother your daughter, you can, of

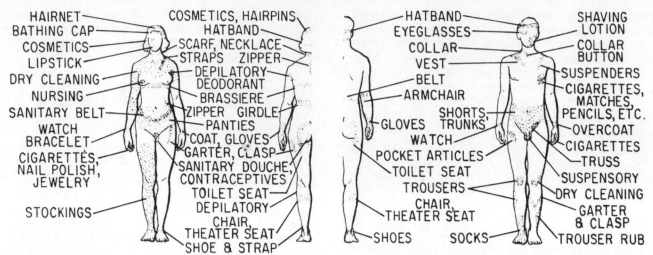

Areas, causes of dermatitis due to allergy or irritation.

course, find other ways of getting its nutrients into her system.

One way to study such a case is to withdraw all of the suspected foods. If the sniffles and sneezes stop, then you can cautiously begin adding the foods, one at a time and for a week or two, until you form a workable knowledge of which ones she can eat in moderation, and which ones she had better avoid entirely.

Please write about asthma. My wife has it. We have consulted several doctors, have gone to Phoenix and Honolulu for the climate, but there has been virtually no relief.

Asthma, difficulty in breathing, results from a number of causes.

What we might call true asthma is a constriction of the bronchial tubes. Air gets into the lungs, but has considerable difficulty in getting out.

Since a sufferer can't get a full supply of air into the lungs until the old air has been expelled, he or she wheezes and struggles for breath.

This closing off (in part) of the bronchial tubes may be muscular spasm, or a swelling of the tissues of the bronchial tubes.

A change of climate is often tried for asthma. There's the natural temptation to say, "Perhaps the air somewhere else will be easier to breathe."

As a matter of fact, such a change many times does help; other times it is a dismal disappointment. Why? Because the two main causes of true asthma are allergy and emotional disturbances.

If the allergy is related to something commonly in the atmosphere of one locality, moving to another climate can give astonishing relief. Conversely, if the allergy involves house dust, food, animal danders, molds, feathers or any of a multitude of other possibilities, another climate won't be the answer.

Also it is close to being axiomatic that the emotions, while not necessarily or even usually the basic cause, will have a strong effect on asthmatic attacks, especially in children. Comfortably at rest, a patient may breathe easily, yet if a strong emotional surge strikes — anger, fear, anxiety, annoyance, frustration, etc. — the asthma comes on again.

What can we do to relieve asthma?

First — and this is not always easy — we must eliminate, or at any rate evaluate, conditions which simulate asthma: Emphysema, scarring of lung tissue, heart disease, and, certainly, any chronic infection which may be inflaming the breathing passages. The first two may permit little improvement; the latter two may yield considerably under medication.

Where none of these is involved, and particularly when the asthma has been present through much of the patient's lifetime, what can we do about true asthma?

Smoking is absolutely taboo.

If the patient is extremely overweight, reduce. Obesity can intensify asthma.

The most promising source of relief is finding what allergies may be present. Just as a "food diary" is an excellent way of tracking down some allergies, you should also keep a careful record of events that precede asthma attacks.

More than food can be involved. Is the asthma seasonal, like hay fever? Does it occur when one is cleaning house? It may be a dust sensitivity.

Attacks can be triggered by medicines, animal danders, cosmetics. Give special attention to such things if the asthma developed after the age of 30 or so; food allergies are more likely to be apparent early in life.

A series of sensitivity (skin) tests can speed up the search for allergens.

Drugs can be given by mouth, inhalation, or in the form of suppositories to relieve the spasm of the bronchial tubes. If they don't relieve the asthma entirely, at least they make the patient more comfortable.

Judicious use of steroids (cortisone and its derivatives) often is helpful.

Will you please give me some information on asthma, emphysema, and fungus of the lung, or are they all the same thing?

These three are entirely different ailments, although they may have similar symptoms. It is also possible for more than one to be present at the same time.

Asthma interferes with breathing because the bronchial tubes become constricted, making it difficult to get air through the small space. That's why the patient wheezes.

Emphysema is quite a different problem. The bronchial tubes are open, but the air cells of the lung have lost their elasticity, and can't accept or push out air in sufficient quantity. There is no drug that will restore the elasticity.

Finally, fungus (viz. histoplasmosis) is one of the organisms which can infect the lungs. (Bacteria, such as the tuberculosis germ and various kinds of viruses, also cause lung infections.)

It is possible for fungus (or other) infections to contribute to emphysema. The infections damage the lung tissues and the result is scar tissue and hence loss of some elasticity.

Severe asthma, over a period of many years, can have its share in bringing on emphysema, by putting excessive and continued strain on the lung tissues. It is possible that your husband may have some of both.

What will stop hay fever? My son, now 24, sometimes nearly smothers to death in damp weather. If he has a cold, his head seems to close completely. Even when he is normal, he coughs and sneezes and his eyes water and swell. He won't go to a specialist. Can you suggest something that will help him?

I'm not sure from the letter whether this condition is only hay fever, or whether it is an allergy which occurs other than in the autumn.

The answers, however, are the same. There are three things that can be done:

1. De-sensitization shots. (For real hay fever, there are injections to help the person tolerate various pollens in the air. For other allergies, different de-sensitizing materials must be added.)

2. Taking antihistamines to ease the symptoms while an attack is in progress.

3. Going to some other climate when the attacks occur. This isn't always practical, of course. In addition, you have to find a place where the offending pollens or other such materials are not present.

There are two main methods of de-sensitization. One is to give a series of injections, starting about six months before the allergy season begins, and gradually increasing the doses.

The other is year-round, giving the injections about once a month to keep tolerance up permanently.

It's a puzzle to me why a young man suffering so severely from allergy should refuse to go to a specialist (an allergist, in this instance).

My doctor tells me that urticaria is causing my hives, but he hasn't been able to cure it. Medicine gives me relief, but pretty soon the trouble starts again. He said he thought diet might help me, but he hasn't given me a diet.

Urticaria is a five-cylinder word for hives, a red, splotchy, itchy outbreak on the skin. The cause: Allergy of some sort.

The allergy may be sensitivity to something you eat, or touch, or something in the air.

Your doctor evidently suspects that in your case it is something you eat, which could account for his mention of diet. But until he (or you) can find out what is bothering you, you won't know what to leave out of your diet.

Watch what you eat or touch. Urticaria usually breaks out fairly soon after contact, sometimes within 10 or 20 minutes.

The medication you have been using is probably an antihistamine drug which usually gives quick relief but cannot "cure" you. Cure depends on avoiding whatever bothers you, or in some cases having desensitization treatment by an allergist.

I swim at the Y.W.C.A. It is good exercise and seems to help a bad back.

My problem is that as soon as I leave the water I start sneezing. My nose runs, and it is difficult to swallow because it drags at my ears. I have tried nose clips and nose drops, but nothing helps. Have you any suggestion other than giving up swimming?

The culprit in pools is most likely the chlorine used to disinfect the water. You didn't mention smarting eyes, but some folks notice that, too.

I won't recommend giving up swimming, which is a wholesome exercise. The sneezing and irritation are a temporary nuisance but they won't hurt you.

My suggestion is this: Learn to be a good mouth breather. Inhale through the mouth, exhale through the nose. Expert swimmers habitually do this anyway.

Nose drops won't help much if at all. As to nose clips, a little water seems always to get into the nostrils despite them, so proper breathing should give you better results.

Eye, Ear, Nose & Throat

THESE FOUR AREAS of specialization used to be combined in a single medical specialty. In more recent years, care of the eye has become a single specialty, treated by the ophthalmologist, and the other three (which are closely interrelated) by the "E-N-T" or ear-nose-throat specialist.

There is a still more recent tendency for some E-N-T men to specialize particularly on the ear, since ear surgery is becoming both more complicated and more effective.

I do not, in this chapter, try to outline these intricate operations, but I do want to call attention to the fact that they now restore hearing in cases which, a generation ago, were regarded as entirely hopeless.

They cannot correct nerve deafness, when the auditory nerve no longer can transmit sound, but such operations as tympanoplasty, stapedectomy (and a considerable number of variations of it) and other surgeries are well worth while.

The specialist in childhood ear diseases often saves youngsters from growing up with impaired hearing. Earache, and particularly infection (as from "a running ear") deserve prompt attention.

In the eye field, the two foremost problems are, I think, the danger of glaucoma, which so often creeps up without warning and leads to blindness; and questions about cataracts.

Periodic measurement of pressure of the eyeball with a rather simple instrument can give advance warning in time to prevent glaucoma from destroying eyesight.

Cataracts are of increasing importance because, with more folks living longer, more have this trouble.

Fortunately surgery to remove cataracts is highly successful. Fitted with suitable glasses, such folks find their eyesight excellently restored.

Another item in this chapter which I know — from the number of letters sent to me — will be of wide interest is one on the proper precautions to be observed when contact lenses are to be worn. Contacts, with these precautions, can be safe. Without them, they can cause trouble.

The left eye of my small son has begun to turn inward. What should I do?

The time to start correcting strabismus (squint, or faultily-aimed eyes) is as soon as it is noticed.

In the first few weeks of life, the eyes drift in odd directions until the baby begins to learn to focus. That's by the time he is, perhaps, three months old.

But after that, if the eyes don't focus, something is wrong. You refer to your "small son," so I gather that he is beyond the infant stage but still is not very old.

Sometimes treatments can be started as early as the age of 12 months; for the best and surest results, the sooner the better.

The basic cause is unequal tension of the muscles which control the eyes. But the underlying reasons vary: Some hereditary fault, injury, disease, or some defect in vision so that the eyes (perhaps near-sighted or far-sighted) try to compensate for a condition which will respond only to medical help.

If the eyes won't focus, the result is that the child sees two of everything. So he twists his face, squints, tries whatever odd tricks he can think of, to get rid of one of these images. In a matter of several years, Nature may take over and shut off vision in one eye — it is simpler to "see" only one image.

Hence you shouldn't wait, and shouldn't, as some people unfortunately do, wishfully tell yourself that "it will correct itself later," or "there's nothing to do about it anyway."

There IS a lot that can be done about crossed eyes (or eyes that look outward, or up or down, or any way except focusing naturally. If you start soon enough, nearly all of these cases can be corrected. If you wait until the child is 9 or 10, a good many cases no longer can be corrected.

Treatments must, of course, fit the case. In some instances glasses help; sometimes that is sufficient for the whole problem. With some youngsters, one eye is weaker than the other, and an eye patch covering the strong eye forces the weaker eye to go to work until it can operate normally with the other one. Special eye exercises can be very useful. Sometimes surgery is best to adjust the tension of the eye muscles.

I am 73. Recently a blood vessel burst in my eye, and the blood covers most of the white. Will this clear up? Or cause trouble? It has not disturbed my vision yet.

And it won't bother your vision or be dangerous. This appearance of blood in the eye can be frightening, but it looks worse than it is, by far.

At your age the capillaries (very small surface blood vessels) can become unduly fragile, and some slight injury (rubbing the eye, a slight bump, straining from a sneeze, etc.) can rupture one. If your blood pressure is elevated, that may be a factor.

However, this blood will absorb in about 10 days with no harmful after-effects.

Be sure to get ample Vitamin C (citrus juices) and calcium (milk or skim milk is the most plentiful source) in your diet, which may lessen any tendency toward future bleeding.

Please explain cause and treatment for conjunctivitis.

Let's make that plural — causes. Conjunctivitis is inflammation of the outer lining of the eye, or conjunctiva. This can result from several causes. Bacterial infection is one, more often called "pink eye" and highly contagious. Treatment is based on antibiotics and isolation until the infection is subdued.

Other causes include virus infection; allergic irritation, such as hay fever; irritation from wind or dust or bugs; irritation from chemical fumes. Treatment depends on which cause is found. Abuse or overuse of the eyes can be a contributing factor.

I was told it is unwise for anyone with glaucoma to eat certain foods. What is a proper diet?

There is no special diet (and no special food) which will retard or prevent glaucoma. Medication which will remove fluid from the body can be helpful.

Shortly after having bought my daughter (she's 18) a pair of contact lenses, I read an article that says you can go blind from wearing them. Is there any truth in this? Now I am afraid to let her wear them.

Contact lenses have become extremely popular, and it is estimated that 90 per cent are worn because people feel they "look better." Others, such as actors, athletes, and some professional people have more urgent reasons.

Contacts are here to stay. I strongly believe in letting the decision rest with an eye specialist who will consider the real need and the individual's temperament (some folks cannot tolerate them). He will also explain proper use,

HORIZONTAL SECTION OF EYEBALL

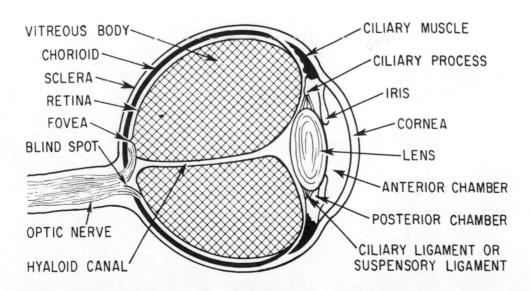

and the necessity for follow-up observation. With simple precautions, contacts are safe.

Anyone wearing contacts should be thoroughly instructed in the right way to insert and remove them; proper cleansing and storage; how long to wear them at a time; and signs of trouble if any develop.

It is essential, in my opinion, that the wearer be checked every six to 12 months to detect any defect in the cornea — the covering of the eyeball. Of course any pain or irritation should be reported to the eye specialist at once.

As to blindness, a recent survey of reports from 1,900 eye specialists on 49,000 patients wearing contacts revealed 14 instances of blindness or loss of vision. These were due to infection, which is why periodic examination is so necessary. If irritation starts, and leads to infection, it must be detected and subdued BEFORE serious damage results.

The foregoing survey also showed that among the 49,000 patients, some complication arose, but was corrected, in 7,600 instances, which bears out the warning I have voiced before: Not everybody can wear contact lenses, and some people can wear them only for a limited time.

What does it mean to see colored halos around street lights at night? Might it be a sign of glaucoma that can cause blindness?

In few words, yes, it might. It also might not. Have your eyes checked! One visit will determine whether you have any cause to worry.

Recently I have been seeing small spots in front of my eyes, like dust specks flying around. What could cause this and how serious is it?

Probably "floaters," meaning tiny particles in the liquid interior of the eyeball. They are quite common and mean that you have joined the rest of us at the age at which they tend to appear. They don't do any harm, except, as I've said before, they can be an awful nuisance sometimes when you are trying to keep your eye on something you are studying through a microscope, or some such chore.

Some people say TV is harmful to the eyes and some say it is not. I have also heard that a small light should be burning between the viewer and the TV set.

No, TV does not harm the eyes. Nor do movies. You don't need a light between you and the TV set, but it is easier on the eyes if there is some illumination in the room.

Is it harmful to use magnifying glasses that are advertised nowadays for close work and reading? I am in my 80's.

No, they're not harmful. They do not, however, correct for other faults in the eyes, such as astigmatism, if they exist.

I am told I have a cataract on one eye. If an operation is necessary, is it serious?

Modern eye anesthetics eliminate pain, and sedatives are used before and after the surgery to take care of the natural nervousness. It's an

The eye is like a camera. Here is a camera with its main portions and portions of the eye that correspond.

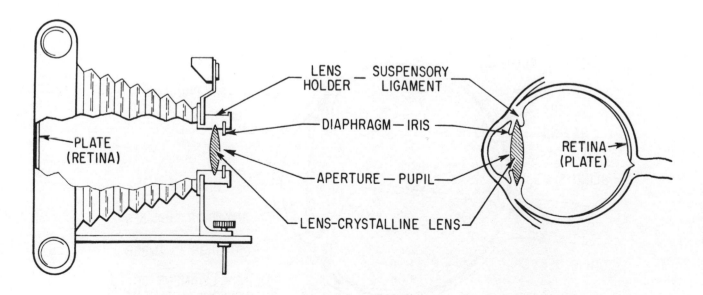

operation demanding precision but I don't think I'd call it a serious one except for that.

Then after the eye is healed, lenses are fitted to direct the light rays to the proper part of the retina, the job done by the natural lens in the eye before the "cataract" clouded it.

The new lenses may be spectacles, or may be contact lenses which are coming into greater use for this purpose.

A cataract actually is a chemical change which causes the lens of the eye to become cloudy, thus gradually preventing sufficient light from passing through.

To date there is no medicine which will correct this.

Cataracts never get better, and if you can't see adequately, surgical removal is the only answer.

I'm often asked when this should be done. It used to be the custom to allow cataracts to "ripen," but these days the decision depends rather on the need for improving vision.

A person who needs to use his eyes for close work should have surgery much sooner than the person who doesn't. I've known plenty of people who, after the operation, vehemently wondered why they had put it off so long.

Are there eye drops which delay the advance of cataracts which already have formed? Will the use of an eye wash morning and night be beneficial?

Eye drops or washes do not retard the progress of cataracts, but can widen the pupil of the eye, admit more light, and hence help vision until the time comes to remove the cataracts surgically.

What is glaucoma, and what causes it? Can anything be done for it?

Glaucoma is an increase in pressure inside the eyeball. As the pressure grows, it not only interferes with vision (it can narrow the field of vision, make it foggy, with halos around lights and so on) but in some cases it causes a dull ache in eyes or the head.

Untreated, it can result in blindness. It is probably the greatest single cause of blindness.

But when treated — that's a happier story. Very often glaucoma can be arrested. The earlier the treatment, the better. Various drugs, drops in the eyes, changes in living habits to reduce tension, sometimes surgery to relieve the pressure — all of these methods and combinations of them are saving people's eyes every day.

Glaucoma is a disease that isn't often found until after the age of 40, or sometimes quite a bit later. Women are affected more than men.

The cause isn't always known. It may be a secondary result of some other eye ailment, but usually is related to circulation changes in the eye.

Glaucoma may come on suddenly and painfully, as an acute case. It may deceptively creep up gradually and quietly, with few or no symptoms you can recognize.

But always the pressure in the eye is too high, which gives us our surest warning. A little instrument called a tonometer can measure this pressure. Once used only by eye specialists, the tonometer is more and more becoming standard equipment of other doctors. When a case is discovered, it is time to consult an eye specialist at once.

What is the ophthalmologist's water provocative test?

It is a test for glaucoma, one of several used to determine this condition. The patient is required to drink a large amount of water in a short time. Changes in pressure within the eyeball then are noted by the ophthalmologist with a special apparatus.

I have a cyst on the edge of my lower eyelid. An ophthalmologist says it must be removed surgically to prevent recurrence. Do you think this is necessary?

Yes, that's the right way. A cyst can be relieved temporarily by puncturing or cutting the top off, but it seals itself and grows again. The only way to get rid of a cyst permanently is to remove it. It is called a chalazion.

What is a perforated ear drum and what precautions are necessary?

A perforated ear drum is one with a hole in it. The ear drum serves two purposes: Transmitting sound vibrations to the middle ear; and, at the same time, keeping infection out.

A chronic infection is the usual cause of a perforated ear drum. Therefore the first question is whether this infection can be subdued, and the second is how to keep further infection out.

If the ear canal is dry (no drainage from it) little need be done except to keep dirt and germs out, and to avoid letting water get into the ear, which also might introduce infection.

A cotton plug is helpful to prevent dust from blowing into the ear. Swimming is, of course, taboo. Avoid getting water in the ear while taking a bath or shower.

If there is drainage, you should have an ear specialist's advice on necessary treatment. If the infection cannot be conquered, a drop or two of rubbing alcohol, full strength (or diluted to half, if full strength is irritating) tends to dry the canal and ward off secondary infection. Hydrogen peroxide, full strength or diluted one-third, may also be used.

Under some circumstances tympanoplasty (surgical reconstruction of the ear drum) is possible. It may or may not improve your hearing.

Please write on nerve deafness, what causes it and whether I can be helped by hearing aids.

Nerve deafness — impairment of the nerves which carry sound impulses from the ears to the brain — can be from injury, from infection, and sometimes from a hereditary fault.

If the nerves lose their ability entirely, nothing can be done. But when the nerves, while less sensitive, still can react to some degree, then hearing aids can help, simply by amplifying sounds to a greater volume.

There are also hearing aids of a special type fitting on the mastoid process and thus creating bone conduction.

Periodically my ear forms a crust inside which seems to peel off but feels quite sore underneath. There is also some swelling toward the outside. I would like your opinion.

A general guess probably is easy: Some sort of recurrent dermatitis or skin ailment. A specific diagnosis is something else, however: Is it a fungus, a bacterial infection, or what? My advice, is to consult a dermatologist (skin specialist) or an ear specialist.

As you know, there is a fad among girls of having their ears pierced. I would like to do it but how should I go about it so they won't get infected? Should I have my doctor pierce them, or some other experienced person?

It's been going on for years. With any of the do-it-yourself methods, every so often infection results, which is painful, dangerous and expensive. The only safe method I know is to have your doctor do it, because he knows how to prevent risk of infection. For him it is a simple procedure.

I read that it is now safe for older people to undergo a new type of surgery for deafness, and that such operations have been proven 90 per cent perfect. Is this possible in healthy people of 75?

We have had a great many gains in ear treatment and they have added up to enormous progress over what was possible 10 or 30 years ago. There are quite a few causes and types of impaired hearing. If the nerve is functioning, a variety of operations can help. If the nerve is not functioning, nothing can be done.

So have an ear specialist examine you. He will discuss the possibilities in your case. Today such surgery is perfectly reasonable for persons of 75 even though it was not so reliable a couple of decades ago.

The doctor has diagnosed my daughter's problem as swimmer's ear. At times it is very painful. Is it contagious?

This is usually a fungus infection acquired in lakes, rivers or streams. Not in salt water.

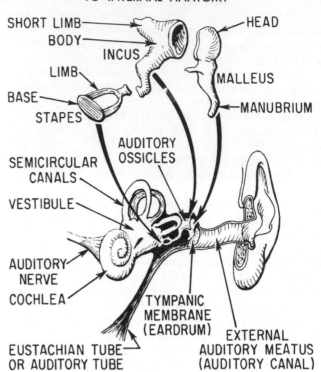

RELATIONSHIP OF EXTERNAL EAR TO INTERNAL ANATOMY

SHORT LIMB
BODY
INCUS
LIMB
BASE
STAPES
HEAD
MALLEUS
MANUBRIUM
AUDITORY OSSICLES
SEMICIRCULAR CANALS
VESTIBULE
AUDITORY NERVE
COCHLEA
TYMPANIC MEMBRANE (EARDRUM)
EUSTACHIAN TUBE OR AUDITORY TUBE
EXTERNAL AUDITORY MEATUS (AUDITORY CANAL)

It is also unlikely to be acquired in a chlorinated swimming pool. No, it is not contagious in the sense of being passed from one person to another. But it must be treated.

I have a hearing problem, but I do not think it has anything to do with volume. If a person speaks distinctly, even if his voice is low, I have no trouble in hearing him. If he has an accent, or drawls or runs his words together or mumbles, I cannot understand even if his voice is loud. Since volume doesn't seem to make much difference, would a hearing aid help?

Maybe one would help. I say "maybe."

It is entirely possible for a person to be deaf to some tones (or sound frequencies) and yet hear others easily. Hearing aids, within limits, can be made to emphasize the frequencies with which you have trouble.

However, I'm not convinced that your problem is quite that simple and I do NOT suggest that you dash off and buy a hearing aid.

Instead, go to an ear specialist who has modern equipment for analyzing hearing defects.

What is the safe way to remove wax from the ears? I have been using a cotton-tip swab but sometimes it makes my ears sore. My college roommate uses a mild solution of hydrogen peroxide to dissolve the wax. Is this a good idea?

I like the old saying, "Never put anything in your ear smaller than your elbow." Washing out excess wax is far safer than trying to dig it out in any manner.

Wax, after all, is a natural protective substance, and should not be removed unless it accumulates to abnormal degree. Soap, water and a washcloth will do all that most of us need, as ordinarily the wax works its way out by itself.

If there is excessive wax and it becomes impacted or hardened, let your doctor or an ear specialist remove it, and advise whether you should thereafter wash some out yourself. A safe method is to use a drop or two of sweet oil or olive oil to soften the wax overnight. Then rinse it out with warm water with a pinch of baking soda added. Use a soft rubber syringe. Do NOT jam it into the ear so that pressure builds up. Let the water flow easily.

Please write about labyrinthitis. At least one-third of my time I'm so dizzy and nauseated I can't do a thing but lie down with my eyes closed.

At times nausea and vomiting grip me so that when it is over even the top of my head is sore.

Labyrinthitis is an irritation of the inner structures of the ear — these structures having a good deal to do with your sense of balance. When your balance is thus upset the nausea is a natural result.

What irritates these inner ear structures? Infection, from bacteria or viruses; or toxic states, as from drugs, certain medications in large quantities, alcohol, tobacco, etc.

For labyrinthitis, treatment is aimed at subduing the underlying infection, of course, along with restriction of salt in the diet, and diuretic drugs to eliminate water and reduce congestion in the critical area. Vertigo pills (medicine to relieve "vertigo" or dizziness) usually help.

I have a deviated septum which my doctor says is a bent or distorted partition between the nostrils. I have difficulty in breathing, a post-nasal drip and a sinus condition.

Is there some cure by medication, or should the partition be taken out?

The nasal septum consists of cartilage, hence can be bent or "deviated" in varying shapes and degrees.

A minor deviation may be of little or no consequence; when the septum is bent enough to interfere with breathing and drainage (causing a post-nasal drip and contributing to sinus trouble) that's another matter.

Can medication correct the bent cartilage? No! This is not to say that some medication may not help in certain phases of treatment, but it can't alter the shape of that septum.

It is usually wise to try some other measures before resorting to surgery, unless the septum is so severely deviated that anything less than surgery is obviously doomed to fail.

The first and most frequent — and the most often ignored by the patient — measure for relief is to give up smoking.

The distorted septum narrows the airway in one side of the nose, and sometimes both. Smoking irritates the membranes and the congestion and swelling still further narrow the airway.

Stopping this irritation (the smoking) and giving the swollen membranes enough time to shrink to normal may be enough to let you breathe easily.

I frequently get serious nosebleeds. They come on suddenly and last a while. What can I do?

The nose usually bleeds from an area on the septum near the nostrils. For this there are two principal reasons. First, the blood vessels are close to the surface, and in some individuals may be more fragile.

Second, an ulcer may have formed — it needn't be large or painful, yet under the circumstances it can cause repeated bleeding. A clot forms, then breaks loose and you have another nosebleed.

First aid is pressure on the nose, or better yet, pack cotton into the nostril, taking care to leave some sticking out, so it can be removed when necessary.

Sit with your head tilted a bit forward — I don't mean with it down at your knees. Don't lie down, because then the blood can run into your throat, and you have no way of knowing when the bleeding has stopped.

Don't remove the packing too soon, as the clot, just being formed, may be dislodged.

For a more permanent answer, have a physician inspect the inside of your nostrils to learn whether you have this bleeding from just one or both sides.

An ulcer can be cauterized, which seals the place from which you have the bleeding. If there is no ulcer, but the point at which the bleeding occurs can be identified, cauterizing that area can also ward off future bleeding. Bleeding can occur higher in the nostrils and the spot may not be accessible by the methods mentioned. In such an instance, special packing by a physician is essential.

Please discuss the cause and remedy for laryngitis.

If you'll make that plural — causes and remedies — we'll get somewhere. Laryngitis is irritation or swelling of the tissues of the larynx, or "voice box," which includes the vocal cords or false vocal cords.

Acute laryngitis is the kind that usually stems from a common cold. The throat is sore.

RELATIONSHIP OF PARTS OF THE RESPIRATORY SYSTEM

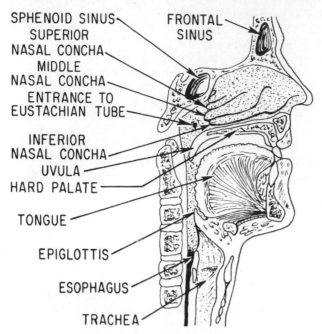

SPHENOID SINUS
FRONTAL SINUS
SUPERIOR NASAL CONCHA
MIDDLE NASAL CONCHA
ENTRANCE TO EUSTACHIAN TUBE
INFERIOR NASAL CONCHA
UVULA
HARD PALATE
TONGUE
EPIGLOTTIS
ESOPHAGUS
TRACHEA

Cross-sectional drawing of the face and neck, depicting nasal, oral and tracheal portions of respiratory tract.

There's hoarseness, often a cough. Smoke, dust or fumes may also cause laryngitis.

That type of laryngitis subsides quickly when the original cause — the cold or exposure to irritants — clears up.

When laryngitis hangs on — and let's say that means anything beyond two weeks — it's time to look for some other cause.

Of course laryngitis may be prolonged if a person persists in smoking. Remedy: Stop smoking. If laryngitis doesn't subside then, consult your doctor.

Singers and speakers can develop "speaker's nodes," or go hoarse, or even lose their voices. For this, the first and urgent treatment is rest for the weary, irritated larynx. Remaining silent for a number of days may be necessary.

We must always, when laryngitis hangs on, consider the possibility of a growth, a benign tumor or, more perilous, a malignant one. Cancer of the larynx is not uncommon, so any lump or growth there should be examined by biopsy, for immediate removal if it is malignant.

Four out of five malignant cases, when discovered soon, are cured successfully. Only one in five is cured if it is allowed to spread to the lymph glands. Can you think of a better reason for having your doctor take a look if you have hoarseness that lasts two weeks or more?

What causes enlarged tonsils and why should they be removed? There is no infection.

Do enlarged tonsils cause infection later if left in?

Tonsils are part of the lymphatic system, which combats infection, but these gland-like structures, with deep crevices, can themselves become chronically infected.

Acute, frequent attacks of tonsillitis, or recurring ear infections, are good reasons for removing infected tonsils. The latter — ear infections — are a dangerous complication which can lead to perforated ear drums, defective hearing or chronic mastoid disease.

In my experience many recurring ear infections have been eliminated by tonsillectomy and I regard it as the most important indication for surgery.

There is variation in the size of tonsils. They may be as small as beans or as large as walnuts, even touching each other. Adenoids also vary, and can interfere with breathing. Mouth-breathing, caused by such enlargement, is valid reason for removal.

We should remember, however, that tonsils tend to become smaller with age. At times they can be quite prominent at age two or three, remain large for several years and then subside, unless chronic infection causes them to remain large.

Advent of the antibiotics has been an important factor. These drugs rapidly subdue acute infections and diminish the frequency of recurrence. In this regard some tonsils are safely and properly allowed to remain today, whereas a generation ago they would have been so infected as to make removal the only wise course.

I wish you would write about bronchiectasis.

This is a disorder of the bronchial tubes, which become dilated (perhaps only in certain areas) and infected. The dilation allows a puddling of mucus and pus. The result is a chronic cough with foul-smelling phlegm. Bronchiectasis also is the commonest cause of blood-tinged sputum. (This condition also can, obviously, be a factor in bad breath.)

Cough, examination of the lungs and the patient's history give ready clues to the presence of bronchiectasis. Duration of the cough, when it started, and the sounds from the lungs are all indicative.

The most specific proof, however, rests in X-ray studies. An iodized oil is instilled into the bronchial system to make the dilated tubes clearly visible.

Bronchiectasis can affect the young as well as the old, and the in-betweens, but keep in mind that smoking aggravates the situation.

Basic treatment consists of the use of antibiotics to subdue infection and measures to help drainage of the clogged tubes. Inverted posture, that is with the shoulders lower than the hips, helps drainage of the phlegm. Drugs to loosen the sticky secretions also are effective in clearing the bronchial tubes.

Digestive & Urinary Disorders

GENERALIZATIONS ABOUT ailments of the digestive and urinary tracts are most difficult. A "gassy stomach" may involve ulcers, gastritis, gall bladder disease — or only something as simple as "air-swallowing."

Pain can mean most of the aforementioned ailments, or be only a muscle spasm, or it can be a heart attack, which is one of the things to suspect when "acute indigestion" occurs. "Indigestion" may mean organic ailments, food allergies, nervous tension for some folks.

The same ambiguity applies to single urinary symptoms. Frequent urination can mean diabetes, kidney disease, bladder infection. Or, again, it can be just nerves. But pus or blood require medical attention.

Therefore, while this chapter may not be the gayest literature in the world, I genuinely do suggest reading it rather carefully, because some knowledge of the stomach, duodenum, gall bladder and urinary system is pretty likely to be useful, soon or late, to almost anyone.

What relation does hiatal hernia have to an ordinary hernia or "rupture"?

Virtually none. Your diaphragm divides the thoracic or chest cavity from the abdominal cavity.

As you swallow food, it passes through the esophagus or gullet. To reach the stomach, it must get past the diaphragm. Nature provides a small opening in the diaphragm for this purpose. Normally it fits snugly and neatly.

But if the aperture becomes slightly enlarged — that is where the rupture or hernia aspect enters in — there can be chafing and irritation. A little of the lower gullet or the uppermost part of the stomach can force its way through the gap, and be excrutiatingly painful, like an ulcer. Or some of the stomach juices can escape into the esophagus and irritate, or cause burning or a "sour rising." The ailment sometimes can interfere with swallowing.

Since the pain so much resembles an ulcer, in earlier years it was often so diagnosed. Today, with X-ray and with more knowledge of hiatal hernia, this error is disappearing.

The treatment, in many respects, is like ulcer treatment: Bland diet, antacids in appropriate cases, sometimes other medication. In addition, a stout person should lose weight — fat in the abdomen tends to push the stomach upward and cause trouble.

One clue is that hiatal hernia many times affects a person when lying down, not when standing up. Why? Gravity draws the stomach down and away from the opening when he stands up. Therefore some patients benefit greatly by raising the head of the bed four or six inches with blocks of wood, so they can sleep more comfortably.

These conservative methods of treatment prove satisfactory in the great majority of cases. Sometimes surgery is required, but it is rarely suggested until the other methods have been tried.

The ailment goes under a variety of names: Hiatal or hiatus hernia; upside down stomach; or esophageal hernia.

Two years ago my husband was hospitalized with bleeding ulcers, but no pain. Since then he has not been bothered until last winter when he had severe pain but no bleeding. X-rays showed a duodenal ulcer plus a shallow gastric ulcer.

Our doctor wanted to operate, saying this stomach or gastric ulcer could become cancerous. My husband then went to an internist who said no, that because of the location and small size it would not become cancerous. Now we don't know what to do.

If this ulcer becomes cancerous, or if it doesn't but becomes so troublesome that it has to be removed anyway, then the first doctor is right.

But if it calms down and heals, then the second doctor is right.

I would be most careful to have continued examinations to watch this ulcer.

Duodenal ulcers rarely are malignant. Gastric (or stomach) ulcers have a much higher incidence of cancer, so when an ulcer is in the stomach rather than duodenum, that's the time to play safe.

X-rays taken periodically, to see whether the ulcer is getting bigger or smaller, are an important safeguard.

It is most certainly wrong to think that all gastric ulcers become cancerous.

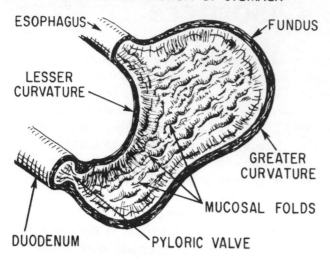

LONGITUDINAL SECTION OF STOMACH

ESOPHAGUS

FUNDUS

LESSER CURVATURE

GREATER CURVATURE

MUCOSAL FOLDS

DUODENUM

PYLORIC VALVE

What is the treatment for duodenal ulcers? What does the "duodenal" mean? Is surgery usually necessary?

The exact cause of duodenal ulcers is not known, although many of the factors involved are very well known.

The duodenum is a short segment just below the stomach — the connection, indeed, to the small intestine. For whatever reason, ulcers (or sores) are likely to form there.

Smoking, nervous tension, heavy drinking all are known to play a part in causing these ulcers. Once the ulcer forms, spicy foods, tension, excessive motility all keep the ulcer irritated.

Therefore a bland diet is prescribed. When the ulcer has periods of hurting, milk or cream or small portions of other bland foods tend to protect it and relieve the pain.

"Motility" relates to the motion of the intestine. Stress or anything else which increases this, adds that much irritation of the ulcer. Spicy foods and smoking — smoking, most decidedly — increase the motility and the release of acid juices which also irritate.

Surgery occasionally is necessary, but it is always a last resort, and may bring new problems in its wake — including new ulcers.

Medications to calm the nerves, to retard intestinal motility, and to reduce the acidity of digestive juices often help.

As to alcohol, doctors are divided. Some prohibit all drinking. Some permit a limited amount if it seems to sedate the patient. But all oppose anything resembling heavy drinking.

X-rays showed I had an ulcer in the pyloric canal. After going on a strict diet I had more X-rays two months later, showing the ulcer had healed. Is it possible for an ulcer to heal that soon? And why does the pain still remain? My doctor says scars can cause as much pain as an ulcer. Would you explain?

Yes, an ulcer can heal that soon, but the puckering of the scar can, in some cases, put strain on tender areas. There may be an element of spasm of the pylorus which can cause pain.

I sincerely hope that they will let a psychiatrist do a thorough job of analysis.

Is flatulence a subject that doctors won't discuss? Surely the medical profession can prescribe at least relief if not cure — neither digestion tablets nor baking soda is effective with me.

The average doctor (and include me) isn't too happy about trying to offer a quick, easy remedy for flatulence. Or let's use a simpler word: Gas.

The answer for some people is so simple that they can't believe it: Don't swallow air! Babies do it. That's why we burp them. Some adults unconsciously acquire the habit of swallowing air. Then they burp.

They tend to swallow air in quantity as they eat or drink. This can be overcome by eating and drinking slowly, and never gulping. There is no pill, no medicine that will prevent air-swallowing.

Where more serious underlying causes contribute, there will be other signs. Ulcers, gastritis, gall bladder disease, hiatal hernia and so on, will make themselves known. But professional diagnosis is important because these complaints require effective treatment. And to treat effectively, you have to be sure of the trouble.

What are the symptoms of gall bladder disease? I have had a pain in my right side by my ribs and below my breast.

I was X-rayed and my doctor said my gall bladder looked all right and he thought it was nerves. Could nerves cause this constant pain?

The usual signs of chronic gall bladder disease include discomfort in the upper right abdomen (but sometimes even in the back); flatulence or (gaseousness); intolerance of fatty foods; general digestive upset. Yet sometimes gall stones cause no symptoms at all.

Since X-ray shows your gall bladder to be functioning properly, it is time to look for other ailments with similar symptoms. Some possibilities are ulcers, kidney disease, or even neuralgia attacking between the ribs.

Yes, even nerves can play tricks like this on you. Spasm at the outlet of the stomach, a not uncommon condition, can at times cause continuing pain. A spastic colon, with cramping, likewise can be due to nerves.

I had an attack of gall bladder trouble and surgery was advised, but I have been feeling so well lately that I hate to be cut unless an-

other attack arises. What danger is involved in not having the operation?

I presume that X-rays showed either gallstones or a gall bladder which is not functioning. Since surgery was recommended, I take it that your age and general fitness are satisfactory — and if you need an operation, the time to have it is when you are physically in good shape.

The risks of putting it off? First, the likelihood of further attacks of gall bladder colic. There was a reason for the first attack; the potential reasons are still there.

Or a gallstone might plug one of the ducts and cause jaundice. Or, with or without that occurring, you could develop empyema (pus in the gall bladder) and surgery might then be mandatory no matter how you feel. Cancer of the gall bladder can also occur.

All of the foregoing are serious complications. Since surgery was recommended have it done and be rid of the danger.

Please discuss a dropped kidney. Is surgery to suspend the kidney serious? Is wearing a girdle (advised by my doctor) any great help? I am a woman of 50 and thin — 90 pounds.

The dropped or "floating" kidney, as it is sometimes called, doesn't always require surgery. In fact, the kidneys are intended to do a little floating around by Nature. They change position slightly when we shift from an upright to a prone position.

The kidneys are supported in part by a surrounding pad of fat. Lean folks like you, without so much "padding," are more likely to have excessive mobility of the kidneys.

Whether anything at all needs to be done depends on the amount of movement, on whether there is any discomfort, and most of all on whether there is any kinking of the ureter (the outlet from the kidneys).

Frequently a snug support (a girdle, in this instance) will help. In some cases, however, surgery may be necessary. This is a major operation but it is not an uncommon one and not to be feared. It is not necessary to cut into the kidney itself, nor into the lining of the abdomen. The approach is through the back, and the supporting tissues of the kidney are drawn snug enough to prevent more than the ordinary amount of movement.

I have had several recent attacks from a kidney stone about the size of a pea. The doctors tell me it cannot be dissolved, that it is too large to pass by itself.

The attacks were extremely painful at the time but after a shot of some relaxing drug I was fine again. However, the doctors recommended surgery or else the kidney may be irreparably damaged.

I understand you have stated that kidney stones CAN be dissolved.

Yes, I wrote that, and it is true. I said that some kidney stones can be dissolved. I did not say that all can.

There are different kinds of kidney stones. Some dissolve; some don't. The size also is important. When a stone, because of size or chemical type, will not dissolve, then have it out surgically.

My son, 40, suffers from kidney stones. What causes them? Would a special diet help?

Kidney stones form basically because the urine becomes too highly saturated with certain chemicals — urates, oxalates and phosphates are among them. Then they begin precipitating out as solids, and become "stones." (There are other technicalities involved, but that's essentially it.)

Drinking lots of water to keep the urine dilute is important in preventing more stones. A change in diet also can help, but must be chosen on the basis of study of the chemical content of the stones. This may be done also to increase or reduce the acidity of the urine, but here again you need expert guidance to know which way to change.

My daughter is three and has always complained of a crampy stomach. Six months ago I noticed that she was going to the bathroom frequently and drinking excessive amounts of water.

THE GALL BLADDER

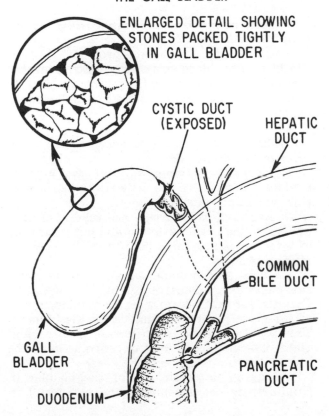

ENLARGED DETAIL SHOWING STONES PACKED TIGHTLY IN GALL BLADDER

CYSTIC DUCT (EXPOSED)

HEPATIC DUCT

COMMON BILE DUCT

GALL BLADDER

PANCREATIC DUCT

DUODENUM

The doctor examined her and found pus in the urine. He began giving her medication but said tests showed quite a bit of pus still, so he X-rayed the kidneys and said the left one is not functioning properly.

He wants me to take her to a urologist and I have made an appointment. Our doctor said there was a possibility of removal of the kidney but that the operation is not serious and that it is good that it was found early.

Could she live a normal life with the kidney removed? Would she have to be under medication the rest of her life?

It sounds as though this youngster has some congenital defect in the left kidney which is conducive to recurrent infections.

You can be sure that a urologist, a specialist in this field, will not remove a kidney unless it is absolutely necessary. There are instances when it is.

Yes, people get along very well with one kidney (note that this is true of a twin who gives one kidney to be transplanted when the brother or sister loses both kidneys.) A single kidney tends to enlarge, to take over the work formerly done by both.

Once the diseased kidney is removed, there would be no necessity for continuing medication, assuming (as appears to be the case) that the other kidney is normal.

There is great risk in a chronically infected kidney. Further danger is that infection in one eventually can spread to the other. There is very good reason for removing a kidney when infection cannot be cleared up permanently, especially if there is some anatomical defect.

What could cause seminal fluid to be clouded with blood?

Usually it's a prostate problem. Have it checked. The blood may originate from the seminal vesicles (a reservoir structure for the fluid) which may be congested or inflamed. It usually is not serious.

What are the causes of acute cystitis, and what is the prognosis?

Cystitis is inflammation of the urinary bladder. Women are particularly vulnerable to this type of an infection.

Acute cases as a rule are readily cleared up. But urine examination to find out what type of infection is present is helpful in choosing the right treatment.

Where the trouble persists or becomes chronic, more extensive testing is advisable. Cystitis, for example, may be a secondary result of infection higher up, that is, in the kidneys. This type of cystitis is likely to be chronic, and quite reasonably will tend to continue until the kidney trouble is corrected.

Sagging or stretching of the bladder in childbirth is not uncommon and can result in

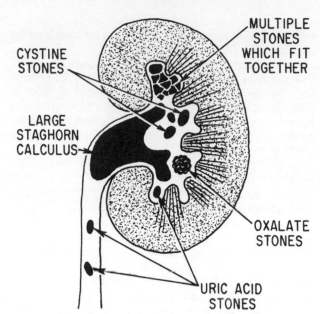

Cross-section drawing of kidney showing various types of kidney stones (calculi) and where they occur. Oxalate and phosphate stones are commonest. Latter type occur frequently in the presence of kidney infection.

incomplete urination and hence some "puddling" in the bladder. This, of course, provides a good medium in which germs can grow. In marked cases of such sagging (called cystocele) a plastic operation may be advisable to support the bladder back in normal position.

In still other cases visual examination of the inside of the bladder by means of a cystoscope may be necessary, to see whether ulceration of the bladder wall may have developed, or polyps or some other growth. Stones, too, can contribute to infection by setting up irritation.

I had a bladder infection which my doctor cleared up with antibiotics but I was still having trouble with the urethra and he sent me to a urologist who has given me four dilating treatments. He said unless it gets too painful I can wait three months before taking the next treatment. I am becoming discouraged.

Discouraged? Why? Signs of progress appear to be unmistakable. I grant that these troubles often take time, but reaching a point at which treatments are three months apart indicates headway.

Bladder infections may often affect the urethra, or tube which drains the bladder. Sometimes there is scarring which partially blocks it, and gradual dilation corrects this. In others, vaginitis related to menopause or other causes can irritate the urethra.

What is uremic poisoning?

It results from faulty functioning of the kidneys. Uric acid and certain nitrogen compounds are wastes which the kidneys filter out and — normally — discharge in urine. When something prevents removal of these toxic materials, poisoning results.

About half an hour after eating, I developed such a severe pain in my lower right side that I could no longer drive.

At the hospital it was diagnosed as renal colic. After an injection and a night in the hospital, I was discharged as in A-1 condition. Can you tell me what brought on this terrible and sudden attack?

Renal (kidney) colic is a very severe pain — as you have learned — caused by the passage of a kidney stone or small blood clots through the ureter, the tube from the kidneys to the bladder. Usually it is a tiny stone or "gravel."

The occurrence is notoriously painful, but once the stone or clot has passed through into the bladder, there is relief. The pain is from the stone being forced through the ureter which is a slender tube. (Very small stones may pass through without pain.)

Once you have had such an attack, the wise thing is to have X-ray or other examination to determine whether stones are still present in the urinary tract. Depending on what he finds, your doctor may adjust your diet or take other measures (especially urging you to drink plenty of fluids, to keep the urine dilute) to discourage formation of more stones.

My husband must have his prostate removed. Will this destroy his sex life?

Usually not, but many men erroneously think that it will. Since the emotions play such a strong role, having this idea can, at least for a time, cause trouble. There is no reason why the operation should disturb sexual activity.

Please explain gastritis, its causes, symptoms and treatment.

Gastritis is a general term meaning that the gastric area — the stomach — is inflamed.

There may be pain, or there may just be a feeling of fullness or pressure. Headache, nausea, vomiting, may follow. Diarrhea is possible.

Treatment depends on the cause. If caused by acids or corrosive chemicals, immediate treatment is required to neutralize them as well as to wash them out of the stomach.

Hiatal hernia (which involves a portion of the stomach being forced through an aperture in the diaphragm) causes that portion of the stomach to be subject to irritation and inflammation. That's gastritis of one type.

Food poisoning, spoiled food, or other poisons and irritants can cause gastritis. Infection, and overproduction of stomach acid are other causes. Alcohol, especially on an empty stomach, is a very common cause. A bland, soft diet usually solves the difficulty in a short time.

The prime question, with gastritis, is "What's inflaming the stomach?" Then the answer is usually readily apparent from a good history of the patient.

After taking an enema I can't have a normal movement for days so I have to take a laxative. Then I fill up with gas and the only way I can get rid of it is to take another laxative, thus forming a vicious circle.

That is one of the misunderstood things about enemas (which occasionally, of course, are necessary). The enema cleans out the colon. It takes time for the colon to fill up again, before nature is ready for another movement.

I think you will find that you do NOT "have to take a laxative." Just wait another day or so for your natural rhythm to resume.

By taking a laxative, you irritate the intestinal tract, and it is no wonder that you have trouble with gas. It will not harm you to wait a little longer.

What could be the cause of loose bowels or diarrhea in a man aged 48? This has been bothering him for six months. Has anyone else had this trouble?

It has happened many times before. The answers? Colitis, "nervous colon," some chronic infection or infestation of the intestine, cancer (the danger signal of "some change in bowel habits"), a partial obstruction yet non-cancerous. Shall I continue the list, or is this enough to persuade you (or him!) that when this condition develops, there is only one thing to do. Have your doctor begin checking to see which of many possibilities is the cause. And the sooner the better.

What causes diverticulosis and diverticulitis? What are the differences, and the consequences if a sufferer doesn't adhere to careful diet? Can either lead to cancer?

Straining, constipation and probably minor weak places in the intestinal wall appear to be the principal causes of diverticulosis. In the colon or elsewhere an outpouching develops. That's a diverticulum. Diverticulosis means you have a diverticulum. Diverticulitis means that this pouched place has become inflamed and irritated.

No, it's not regarded as leading to cancer. Indeed, in our more advanced years, as many as a quarter to a third of us may have diverticulosis and not even know it.

It is when one of these areas becomes infected and under continued irritation that it may be serious, so it pays to understand it and to keep it from reaching such a stage.

Surgery isn't often needed. Removal of the distressed portion of the colon would be warranted only if serious complications develop — recurrent bleeding, perforation of the colon and the formation of abcess, or stricture

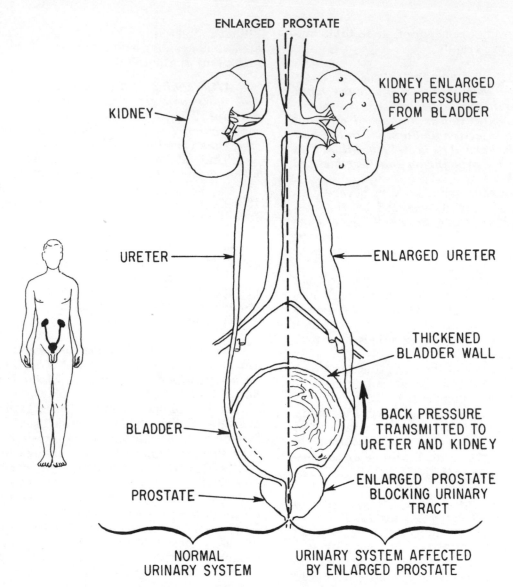

ENLARGED PROSTATE

KIDNEY

KIDNEY ENLARGED
BY PRESSURE
FROM BLADDER

URETER

ENLARGED URETER

THICKENED
BLADDER WALL

BACK PRESSURE
TRANSMITTED TO
URETER AND KIDNEY

BLADDER

PROSTATE

ENLARGED PROSTATE
BLOCKING URINARY
TRACT

NORMAL
URINARY SYSTEM

URINARY SYSTEM AFFECTED
BY ENLARGED PROSTATE

(narrowing) of the colon as a result of repeated attacks and hence formation of scar tissue.

In such cases as do necessitate surgery, it is impossible to say in advance that a bland, non-irritating diet will be mandatory afterward, but in general I would have to say yes, such a diet would be wise. You will be rid of the pouched section, but you will have the scar where the operation and rejoining of the colon was performed and it is only sensible to follow a diet which will give reasonable promise of not irritating that area.

What causes inflammation of the bowel? Why should it recur every few months? I have not been told to follow any particular diet.

Such chronic, recurrent irritation can be caused by ulceration of the colon, or by a variety of germs and parasites. Culture and study of stool samples (to identify any parasites or harmful germs) plus, if possible, direct inspection of the bowel with a proctoscope, to determine the cause and nature of the inflammation, are essential. If parasites or germs are respon-

sible, you have to find out what they are before you can eliminate them. A special diet, unless you know what it is supposed to accomplish, is of no consequence.

Why do some men have prostate trouble and others not? Basically what is the cause?

The exact cause of prostate enlargement is not known, but it occurs in about one-third of men over 60. Symptoms are frequent urination day and night; reduced stream force; hesitancy starting stream and dribbling after. Like fibroids of the uterus in women, the ailment is common but the explanation is elusive. (Incidentally, simple enlargement of the prostate is not cancer. Malignancy may exist, too, but this is coincidence, not cause and effect.)

Many cases are adequately treated by massage of the prostate. Others require surgery, which can range from merely enlarging the central aperture to complete removal of the gland which may be necessary because of cancer. Hormone treatment also is suitable and effective in some cases of prostate cancer.

Growing Old More Happily

M OST PEOPLE COULD grow old more happily, and with better health, if they only would. While this chapter is devoted to various medical problems which beset elderly folks, I want to preface it with some thoughts on the positive rather than negative side.

What can you do to *avoid* some of the troubles which are characteristic of growing older?

Of course, you can't really say that any particular disease is exclusively a disease of age. Rheumatoid arthritis can attack at any age, even in childhood. Heart disease, and even strokes, can afflict the very young. Older folks must look in many chapters of this book, not just one, to find answers about specific diseases, because it is quite impossible to separate the ills associated with age from the ills that also afflict youth and the middle years.

But we DO have to admit that many problems are more likely to occur as we grow older. We can't stop the years in their flight, but we CAN do certain things to keep the years from causing so much trouble.

I would like to steal a remark from the noted Dr. Alton Ochsner on what he calls "early senescence." Of it, he said, "We have become a sedentary people who eat, drink and smoke too much, and exercise too little, only sporadically, or not at all."

This comes as close as anything to telling, in a sentence, what makes people grow old too fast.

Overweight puts more strain on the joints (arthritis), on the heart, on the digestive system. It elevates the blood pressure and increases the risk of a stroke. It increases the risk of diabetes which in turn can affect the heart, the eyes, the legs. And that's just the start of the list.

As for exercise, that plays its part in keeping weight down to normal, but it does much more than that. Regular daily activity keeps joints from stiffening, improves circulation, helps to avert leg cramps. It also is extremely important in keeping the heart in good running order. Repeated experiments with patients with failing hearts and angina pectoris show that exercise can improve their hearts.

I will not belabor the smoking point — cigarets in particular — nor try to list the ways it helps to give up cigarets. I'll just say that the benefits are real. So think it over.

One thing Dr. Ochsner did not stress but I will is the importance of keeping *interested*. The mind as well as the body thrives on use, becomes flabby with idleness. Keep up with the news, keep up with your friends and their activities, read, pursue a hobby. Read new books, bought or borrowed from the library, as well as some of the old ones. Work on committees. Organize card and dance clubs. It is the old person who "just sits" who becomes senile.

So much for things senior citizens can do for themselves. Now a list of items to be kept in mind by people who have elderly folks in the household:

See that their teeth (or dentures) are in useable condition. Difficulty in eating is one reason for poor nutrition. Foods that are easiest to eat are favored to the exclusion of necessary foods.

See that meals are balanced and varied. Pay particular attention to seeing that there is ample protein (lean meat, fish, eggs, cheese), and calcium (a couple of glasses of milk a day, in whatever form), fresh green vegetables, daily citrus or tomato juice.

Have the older person's eyes checked. The person who can't see well is not going to find much interest in reading — not to mention the danger of stumbling or falling just because of poor sight.

What about footwear? Old, floppy slippers are an invitation to a fall. So are slippery floors, throw rugs, loose or torn carpeting, toys or other items cluttering the floor.

Make sure that railings and bannisters are solid. Put a skid-proof safety mat in the bathtub. Install grab bars or other solid hand-holds.

And include the older relative in your life. That doesn't mean that the older person, like the person of any age, doesn't appreciate a little solitude. But the rest of time include the older person in your conversation, plans, hopes, achievements, problems. Many an older person is reluctant to intrude on affairs of "the young folks," but would give anything just to be included, to be "one of the family."

My feet and legs are always cold up to the knees. Could this be due to poor circulation? If so can anything be done to relieve it? I am past 75.

At your age (and sometimes a lot younger, too) coldness can indeed be due to faulty circulation. The underlying cause usually is hardening of the arteries.

Various medications may be effective in improving the circulation, and hence in making you more comfortable. They may not solve the problem totally, but with most of the creeping ailments of age, smart folks do what is possible to minimize the discomforts instead of expecting total cure.

Another helpful measure, and a simple one, is Buerger's Exercises, which I have described before. This is simply a matter of lying on your back, then raising and lowering each leg alternately. Raising each one for one minute, 10 times, often helps. A simple way to say it is upside down bicycle riding.

In some advanced cases, sympathectomy may be in order. This is an operation, and not a risky or complicated one, in which a nerve trunk is cut. The nerve is the one which controls arterial tone. The resultant relaxation of the arteries permits a stronger flow of blood.

Beyond these measures, in some instances a special X-ray study of the arteries can disclose whether any actual obstruction of blood flow is involved, as contrasted to simple reduction of it. In some severe cases of arteriosclerosis, replacement of a portion of an artery with plastic tubing is possible.

I shouldn't forget one more thing, for those to whom it applies. Smokers suffer more because tobacco contracts the surface blood vessels and thus impairs circulation. If you smoke, stop.

Please discuss poor balance in older people. This is entirely different from dizziness. What does the inner ear have to do with it?

First, let's agree that vertigo, or dizziness, DOES have a lot to do with loss of balance. That is where the inner ear is important.

The inner ear contains a set of semicircular canals — chambers filled with fluid. The canals are arranged in different directions and planes. As we change position, the fluid in the canals flows accordingly, and this is how we know, even in the dark, whether we are leaning forward or back, or to either side.

If infection, hardening of the arteries, changes in blood pressure or other factors disrupt the accurate operation of these tiny canals, our sense of balance can be disturbed. We may or may not feel "dizzy," but balance is disturbed.

As for other things which can cause poor balance in an older person (or younger one, at times) and cause one to stumble and sometimes fall, we must consider other senses which we employ to maintain our sense of position.

We use our eyes. Shut your eyes and try to walk in a straight line. You soon wander. Anything that interferes with eyesight also impairs balance — cataracts, lack of correct glasses, dim vision.

Muscular co-ordination is important. Walk sidewise along a hill, and you know you are on a slope because one foot is higher than the other — poor depth perception is the most usual problem of aviators.

I am over 65, and for about two years have had black and blue spots all over my body and arms and legs. I should describe them as broken veins such as might be caused by a severe bruise.

They come and go. Sometimes there is pain but usually not. My regular physician suggested lemon juice in the morning. Could you discuss this?

This doesn't sound like ordinary bruising — although that is something that rather frequently bothers folks who aren't getting enough calcium or Vitamin C in their diet. The lemon juice provides Vitamin C.

It doesn't sound like a matter of broken veins, which would appear primarily in the legs and be associated with a stinging sensation.

This raises a suspicion (from your description) of some form of purpura, or hemorrhaging in the skin or other surface tissues. Purpura may result in a decrease in blood platelets, or special cells in the blood which have to do with clotting.

Drugs, certain toxic conditions, or even allergies can be factors in this. So also can a deficiency in Vitamin C.

If your condition is purpura, and if it is bothersome enough to warrant more elaborate investigation, a complete blood study, including a platelet count and prothrombin time test may provide the necessary clues.

Recently I read that millions of older people have thyroid deficiency, and that in some instances it is so severe that they suffer from emotional problems such as anxiety, depression, etc. Most suffer from fatigue. Is it possible for thyroid deficiency to cause these problems?

What is considered a normal PBI count for a person of 60? Is a count of 3.5 to 5 too low? Does thyroid deficiency affect blood sugar level?

It would be wrong to foster the idea that everybody over 60 ought to fret about the thyroid, because most thyroids, like most brains, stomachs and other organs keep on patiently doing their duty at 60, 70, 80 and 90.

Yet the thyroid can account for varied symptoms if it gets subtly out of whack. It may be overactive, or underactive. Depression, associated with fatigue, dry skin, hair problems and such, can be due to low thyroid output. It is also possible for anxiety and jitters to be the result of a thyroid gland which is overactive.

The normal range of PBI (Protein-bound iodine, which is a splendid measurement of thyroid activity) is 3.5 to 7, in most laboratories, depending on the method used. In the lower range, the patient may benefit from thyroid medication. And yes, thyroid deficiency can be a cause of low blood sugar, but it isn't the only one.

Will you send me the names of some good books on senility? I am nearly 81 and still working and in pretty good health. However I note that some relatives show signs of senility. The prospect of coming mental deterioration is not pleasant and I wonder what I can do to keep my wits to the end.

Senility — in the sense of mental deterioration as age advances — isn't everybody's lot. Judging from your letter, I would say that you have no sign of it, and if you are still working at goin' on 81, you've taken mighty good care of yourself.

Some people begin to go to pieces mentally in their 50's or even earlier. Others keep their wits about them until they are 100 or more.

Why? The possible factors are being studied constantly. The condition of the arteries, particularly those in the brain, or arteries which feed blood to the brain, obviously is important. All sorts of other conditions may have an effect: Emphysema or other respiratory ailments which curtail adequate oxygen; kidney or liver disease or failure; chemical changes, probably in the enzymes of the body, causing weakness of vital organs. Different causes and different combinations of causes exist.

Avoiding senility isn't something that we accomplish after we are old; we do it by maintaining our health all our lives, and remaining active — but not trying to do more than our physical resources will allow. A person with a damaged or weakened heart often adds many years of useful life by being careful not to exceed the amount of activity his heart can support.

No, my friend, I don't think you need any books on how to avoid senility. It appears to me that you must have spent a lifetime doing a good job of that. Just remain interested in life, people and the world around you.

By the way, have you heard about this slogan that someone noticed in a home for old folks? It says:

"Don't begrudge old age. Many are denied it."

What is the usual expectation of recovery from a fractured hip for a woman of 60? How long should it take? The patient is otherwise healthy. Is it necessary to remove the pin for complete recovery?

It used to be that a fractured hip in an older person was a virtual sentence of death. Long weeks or months of immobility in bed led to general deterioration of health and the usual outcome was pneumonia or some similar illness.

Today the picture is entirely different, although it still can be a very serious condition. It depends on the nature of the fracture as well as the age and general condition of the patient. A feeble, elderly person may not be able to tolerate the shock and pain.

For a healthy woman of 60 (that's not

old) the prospects are good. Fractures can occur in various parts of the hip and the use of a pin depends on that.

No, such pins are not necessarily removed, and in some cases may be left permanently.

Once the fracture has been reduced and pin inserted, the patient usually is made to sit up in two or three days. I say "made," because although the change in position may be painful and awkward, it is essential to maintain general health and avoid congestion in lungs and legs. This is an all-important element of recovery.

How long? I suppose you mean the ability to bear weight on the injured hip. Every case is different. Old bones don't mend as rapidly as young ones. However, X-ray shows the progress of the healing process.

Use of crutches or walkers may permit the patient to get around before the leg can support any substantial weight. Sometimes the patient's reluctance to try to get around in that fashion is emotional rather than real — but be guided only by your doctor as to how much urging is warranted, and when.

Since hip fracture is a common home accident, here are a couple of pointers to remember: Initial clue to a fractured hip, besides pain in the hip, is that the foot is usually turned outward. The patient also is unable to raise his heel from the floor while lying on his back.

Leave the patient lying where he is until the doctor or ambulance arrives. The only first aid you can safely give is to keep the patient warm and as comfortable as possible.

What is the best advice for people over 50 who have lived in Florida for 10 years but intend to take a trip north? Our blood is thin. How do we get back to normal?

Blood doesn't get "thin" from living in a warm climate, although that belief is hard to dispel. There is nothing you need to do in advance. You just have to get used to the colder climate when you get there.

Is it safe for a man of 62 with a heart condition to take flu shots? Do the shots elevate blood pressure? Does alcohol in moderation destroy value of the shots?

You are just the type of person who will benefit most from flu shots. With a heart condition you want to avoid serious respiratory disease. The shots won't affect your blood pressure, and alcohol doesn't destroy their value.

My mother's severe back pains have been diagnosed as osteoporosis and the doctor has started her on hormones. She is 74. What is the outlook? Will she likely become bedfast? Is it safe for her to continue her normal activities?

Are fairly long trips in a car safe? Is any special diet helpful?

Osteoporosis is a problem of aging bones. Calcium is gradually lost and the bones become somewhat brittle and porous.

This condition is from three to six times as frequent in women as in men, and is often associated with the hormone changes which accompany menopause.

However, that is not the only possible cause. Disorders of the pituitary, thyroid and adrenal glands can lead to similar upsets in hormone balance. Or osteoporosis may be related to digestive disorders which prevent proper absorption of calcium.

And one other cause: Disuse of bones (as a paralyzed arm or leg) leads to a loss of calcium.

The outlook is not unfavorable with proper treatment, and there is small likelihood of becoming bedfast unless some other problem intervenes.

Since activity encourages strengthening of the bones, a patient should remain active — but should avoid hazardous things because of the risk of a fall and fracture of a brittle bone. Your mother should watch her step on the stairs and slippery floors. And avoid ladders, standing on chairs and that sort of thing. Loose throw rugs are also a menace.

Administration of hormones is a major medical measure, estrogen alone, or estrogen mixed with the male hormone in proper proportions.

Diet is extremely important, and it must be high in protein. Too many older folks, sometimes because of defective teeth or finicky appetites, skimp on meat and other protein foods. Finely ground meat may be easier to eat. Eggs, fish and dairy products also contain protein.

Attention should be paid to a diet that contains plenty of vitamins, and a vitamin supplement, with emphasis on B and C. Calcium may be given either in the form of generous servings of milk, or in tablet form.

As to long automobile rides, there is no objection; however, a pillow at the small of the back may afford considerable comfort.

I am close to 80 years old. A few weeks ago my right arm and leg gave out. I couldn't control them. This only lasted a little while. The doctor told me I had had a stroke. My blood pressure was 172.

I get so weak during the day I can hardly complete my work. Can I do anything to prevent another stroke?

One stroke does not mean that you are bound to have another, but it is only good sense to take reasonable precautions.

Your blood pressure may or may not have had anything to do with your stroke. Some strokes are from a ruptured blood vessel, others from a clogged one. To be on the safe side, medication to reduce your blood pressure may be in order.

A period of weakness is to be expected following a stroke. Fortunately yours was relatively mild. Keep active but do not be in too much of a hurry to regain your strength. It takes time. Don't overdo. Work a bit, rest a bit. Go on living your normal life, but don't expect to do at 80 what you could do at 40. We aren't built that way.

I am 67, in good health and fairly active, but when I go to bed I get a nervous twitch in my leg and have to get up and walk about 300 paces before I can go back and not be bothered for the rest of the night. This happens every night. What can I do?

This sounds like a condition that has been named "jitter legs." We don't know the cause, but it occurs in older persons. It might be some circulatory disturbance. A short walk (of 300 paces or more) before you go to bed might end the problem, although I don't guarantee it. It may be that the trouble refuses to appear until after you have relaxed. Quinine in small doses at bed time may help. The condition is a nuisance but not particularly serious.

My father, aged 77, suffered a mild stroke. Are there exercises that can help his coordination? His left hand and leg are affected but his speech is o.k.

Yes, exercises or other forms of physical therapy are often helpful, especially in milder strokes, but it is impossible to generalize, because cases vary so much.

Your physician. or better yet a rehabilitation center which specializes in such things, can best recommend suitable exercises or other methods of treatment.

Some victims have helped themselves a good deal just by conscientiously doing simple "exercises" using the affected parts. For example, raising and lowering a small weight with the partially-paralyzed arm keeps the muscles toned up and gradually improves coordination so that more complex movements gradually become possible. Don't anticipate much improvement too soon; it isn't easy and it won't bring complete recovery as a rule, but with persistence it will help substantially.

I am a woman of 62. My doctor says I have a fallen bladder. What caused it?

It can occur with age as a result of loss of tissue tone. The supporting tissues may also have been stretched or damaged in childbirth. Not all cases need special attention. The chief problem is infection or irritation when the bladder does not empty completely. If severe, surgery is necessary to provide better support.

An aged parent who has always been gentle and kind — a wonderful companion to a beloved daughter — suffers from arteriosclerosis ("hardening of the arteries") of the brain.

The parent finally has become absolutely indifferent to this daughter, has made cutting remarks, and no longer appears to love or want her. Can you explain what has caused this dreadful change?

Degeneration of the arteries of the brain decreases thinking ability. There may have been

THE BODY VS. THE MIND

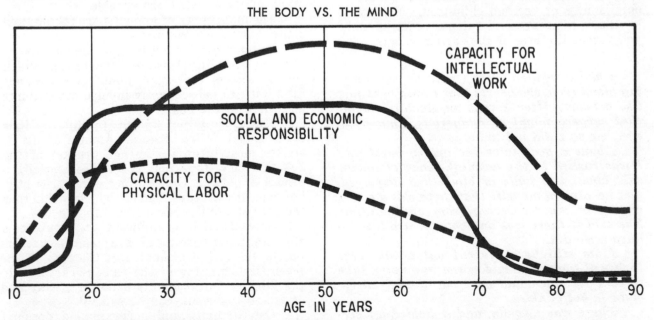

This chart illustrates graphically one of the greatest problems of the aged: the fact that the capacity for intellectual work remains long past the time when other considerations make it easy for him to find a useful place in society. (Copyright, W. B. Saunders, 1949.)

some small strokes; or there may have been only the gradual diminution of blood supply to various areas of the brain.

Brain damage can impair physical response — the patient is slow, shaky, may be paralyzed to a varying extent, perhaps unable to walk.

We can understand such changes and accept them as a form of aging which we are unable to prevent.

But when the brain damage, instead of causing only physical consequences, takes the form of a change in personality, we find it harder to accept. We realize that the paralyzed patient does not walk because she can't — not because she doesn't want to. If some other part of the thinking apparatus — the brain — becomes damaged, we do not always realize that it is the same sort of condition. The reasoning power has been impaired.

Perhaps that will let you bear your troubles more philosophically.

There may or may not be a deep-seated emotional element involved. In some cases, a parent, over the years, becomes accustomed to ruling the household, and telling a child (even when grown up) what to do and how to do it.

When authority passes, as in time it must, to a daughter, there can be resentment on the part of the parent. This is rebellion against the facts of life and old age. But the manifestation sometimes takes the form of lashing out against the daughter.

It means no more than the railing of a little child who may say, "I hate you!" Children do, sometimes, but they learn to control their emotions, and to evaluate life.

An aged person can burst out with the same sort of resentment. It is, after all, a sort of childishness or "second childhood." Try not to let the indifference and cutting remarks make you forget the love of the earlier years.

I had a swollen aorta (main artery carrying blood from the heart) that would beat just like a heart. After X-rays my doctor told me that surgery might be dangerous. That bothered me so I did not undergo it.

About a year later the artery burst and I was rushed to the hospital. Another doctor said about two pints of blood had dispersed, and he advised my wife that there was a slight chance of my recovering from an operation. She said if there was any chance at all, to go ahead. He did.

I am still here. He cut out about eight inches of the artery and sewed in a nylon tube to take its place, and gave me blood transfusions in both ankles.

There was no pain, and it healed up perfectly. I was 81 at the time and am now 86.

Doesn't that provide an answer for older people who wonder about surgery? A decade or two ago a person's age was a serious consideration, but it has been steadily declining in importance.

No single thing has caused this. It is an accumulation of many techniques and methods which have been painstakingly developed to avoid complications. We used to laugh grimly at the statement that "the operation was successful but the patient died." Yet that often was the literal truth. The operation itself succeeded but a complication caused the death. Foreseeing and guarding against such complications is the means by which surgery has become so much safer for older people.

What is rheumatism? How does it differ from arthritis? What is rheumatoid arthritis?

Rheumatism is a word that is gradually going out of use, and it indicates just about whatever the user happens to have in mind, in the way of joint or muscle pain.

Muscle strain is often called rheumatism, for no particularly good reason. Foot strain from weak arches can cause pain in the legs and knees and can be incorrectly called rheumatism. Some others are fibrositis (inflammation of fibrous tissues), often in the back; and various forms of neuralgia, stemming from interference with a nerve.

Arthritis means, or is supposed to mean, inflammation or pain or stiffness in a joint. This includes gout or "gouty arthritis" as well as a number of other forms.

However, arthritis often is used as loosely as rheumatism.

This is not good, because too often people label a pain as being arthritis and put up with it, instead of having an accurate diagnosis. Many of these pains are curable.

The main types of arthritis are rheumatoid arthritis and osteoarthritis.

Rheumatoid arthritis is — or may be — savagely disabling. It is a specific disease, which usually affects the small joints of the hands first, but can subsequently involve other joints anywhere in the body.

The cause is not known. In children it is often called Still's disease. Among adults it strikes most often in the age bracket of the 20's and 30's. It is not, you see, essentially a disease of old age. Unless it is treated promptly, however, it can leave damage which will bother the patient for the rest of his life.

Osteoarthritis is different. It, too, affects the joints, but because of wear and tear. Various injuries, the thickening of the ends of the bones, the thinning of the pads of cartilage in the joints — all gradually make us creaky and stiff, and the result can be painful.

Osteoarthritis, unlike rheumatoid, does not spread from one joint to another, nor does it lead to such crippling.

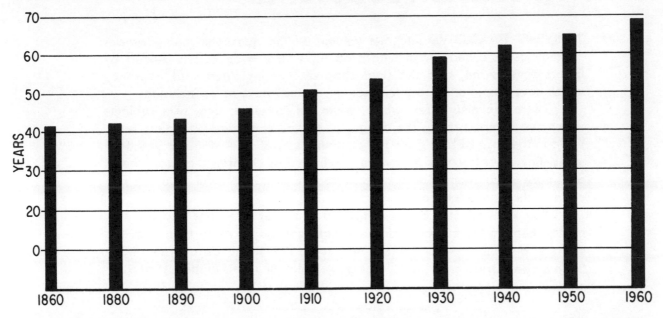

This graph shows constant increase in average life expectancy in the U.S. during period from 1860 to 1960. (Adapted from data furnished by National Office of Vital Statistics.)

I recall reading a comment that a person should "start preventive treatment for arthritis." It startled me as I was under the impression that arthritis could neither be cured nor prevented.

Now I am sure I am developing arthritis, enlarged knuckles, extreme tenderness to pressure. I use my hands a great deal and would be most interested in any preventive treatments available.

You are right in that the disease cannot be cured or prevented, but arthritis can be made more tolerable, and a good deal of disability can be prevented.

Avoiding excessive strain on the joints, yet using them to keep them mobile, moving them to the fullest extent possible, will keep them from "freezing" or becoming stiffer. Keep in mind the difference between using and moving these joints, and exerting them. Aspirin and heat (whether dry heat or warm baths) are a time-tested, reliable methods of easing discomfort. Other medications for the most part depend on supervision by your doctor.

For arthritis, is sodium salicylate beneficial? Is it preferable to buffered types of aspirin? I know someone who takes sodium salicylate tablets but the druggist recommends Vitamin C along with them. Is this necessary?

Of all medications, including cortisone, which can be spectacular for limited periods, the salicylates (aspirin) have proved the most dependable, the safest, and also the least expensive.

Read the labels of the various "aspirin" and related compounds. Mostly they will contain acetylsalicylic acid, and acetophenitidin.

Quite a few will contain caffein, which is a pepper-upper, and also helps conquer some kinds of headaches.

Others will contain a "buffering" material. This is primarily useful in moderating the irritating effect which, some people find, upsets their stomachs. Others have no such trouble. In fact, most of us don't.

How successful is surgery on the hands when they are drawn by rheumatoid arthritis?

I can't give a categorical answer. There are several important factors to consider. One is the patient's general condition, of course. Another is morale. The arthritic process should be inactive for at least six months — it is pointless to try to correct the deformity when the arthritis is still at work and can create further damage.

Surgical correction of the small joints of the fingers is not as successful as of the hand as a whole, or larger joints such as elbow, knee, shoulder.

In some cases arthritis draws the hands into a tightly rigid position. The fingers are permanently bent and immobile, not like a fist, but forward from the large knuckles.

Frequently such hands can be restored to essentially normal appearance. Their usefulness is much improved, but the degree of this depends on the amount of damage, effectiveness of physiotherapy and perseverance of the patient.

General Health Problems

TRYING TO CROWD into one volume all the questions that a reader may ask is a head-scratching problem. I have been largely guided by letters sent to me, and this final chapter contains dozens of questions which have come to me so often that I know they have to be included.

There are also a few which, while not frequent, deal with subjects which need emphasizing: The danger of carbon monoxide poisoning; what to do in the case of burns; the facts about vaccination — too many people still believe that because they were vaccinated as children they don't need any more inoculations. But to keep protection at a high level, boosters are needed through adult life.

You will find also in this chapter a group of questions dealing with mental health. The subject is so vast that I can do no more than skim the surface, but it is important to remind people that tremendous strides have been made in treating mental illness and emotional upsets in the last decade or two.

You say that great advances have been made in treating mental illness, but what are they? What can be done other than sending people to a mental hospital?

Severe psychosis still means hospitalization — but the important advances have been in the field of *keeping* more patients out of the hospital, or in returning hospitalized patients to normal life more quickly.

One great breakthrough was the development of the tranquilizers. From the time of their appearance, we have for the first time been able to curb the terrible overcrowding that used to exist in the hospitals.

For many patients, too upset by anxieties to pay attention to psychiatric therapy, the tranquilizers have meant that tensions could be markedly eased. The patients could begin to look more rationally at their own problems, and begin to solve them.

In other cases, merely allaying anxieties is enough to permit a patient to return to ordinary society without being overcome by the fears and tensions which are the key to so many cases of "mental illness."

Finally, a great many folks, who formerly were destined to be locked up in a mental ward, never have to be hospitalized at all, thanks to tranquilizers.

Another significant advance, not as dramatic as the development of tranquilizers, but of immense importance, is growing recognition by the public at large that emotional illnesses *can* be treated successfully, and the sooner the better.

People are more willing to admit that they are having trouble and need help. Thus diagnosis is made sooner, and treatment begins at an earlier stage instead of being deferred so long that a case becomes chronic and difficult or impossible to treat effectively.

A third important advance is the development, more recently, of the psychic energizers, used for treating various types of severe depression. True depression can leave a patient emotionally drained to the extent of being unable to work or pursue a normal life, and many times there is grave risk of suicide.

Is a nervous breakdown serious? What causes it? Does it ruin one's health? Is hospitalization required?

Nervous breakdown is not a true medical term. It is a catch-all phrase. And sometimes, frankly, it is used because somebody is trying to hide the truth — why, I even know of some people who use "nervous breakdown" when the patient really has tuberculosis. Fantastic, isn't it?

But generally speaking, the term really means an emotional crisis. The patient is unable to cope with some problem or combination of them.

Physical ailments may contribute, and extreme fatigue is one notable condition which is reflected in emotional troubles. However, there may also be good physical health, yet a "nervous breakdown."

Frustration over a job, love or marriage, combined with worry or anxiety over any number of other things are among the frequent causes.

Type and length of treatment depend on the cause. Rest, good nutrition and reassurance, along with helping the patient to look at his problems reasonably and refuse to be panicked by them, will bring an end to many a "nervous breakdown." In some instances psychiatric care may be needed, possibly psychoanalysis.

Once the patient overcomes his problems, or learns how to cope with them, he can be counted as recovered and probably will have no more trouble unless new pressures pile up on him.

When such a "nervous breakdown" patient is referred to a hospital, the inference is that the case is a psychosis, or deep-seated mental illness. "Nervous breakdown" is then too mild a term. It is, in short, a means of evading the use of the term "mental illness." But avoiding the truth is no way to solve our troubles.

When hospitalization is necessary, the extent of the illness is the all-important question. Sometimes only a few days or a few weeks are required to straighten out a case that has not been too-long neglected. On the other hand, some people refuse to face the truth until a case has gotten completely out of hand, and then there is far more danger that the patient may have to remain hospitalized for a long period of time.

As with physical illnesses, so with emotional or mental ones: The sooner they are treated, the greater the prospect of full, rapid recovery.

My husband has been in a mental hospital four times in the last seven years. He has been home now for 13 months and is taking a 100-mg. tablet of a tranquilizer three times a day.

When I suggest that he see a doctor about whether he needs to continue the medication, he says he will just stop taking it himself. I am afraid for him to do that because it might result in a recurrence of his illness. He is listless and sleeps much of the time.

Tranquilizers are much used — and of much value — in relaxing the everyday stresses for people with emotional problems. Sometimes these drugs are the difference between a patient going home or having to stay in the hospital.

I can think of a case or two within my personal experience of patients refusing to take medication of this type with disastrous results.

Most, however, realize the importance of the extra help afforded by the medicine. This is a major factor in recent advances in mental health. We ARE getting more patients home sooner, and keeping them well for longer and longer periods.

I would, therefore, be very much opposed to your husband stopping the medication, or changing the amount of it, without having instructions from a doctor, and preferably from a psychiatrist.

Isn't it possible for him to go back to the hospital to see the doctors there, say every few months? Not to stay, but just a call in the office. You might write to the hospital and ask

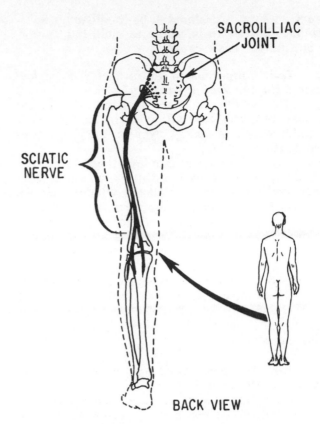

LOCATION OF SCIATIC NERVE

whether a visit would be advisable, or whether there is a clinic or a psychiatrist closer to your home.

What is the best thing to do for sciatica?

The best thing to do for sciatica is, first, to find out what is causing it.

Sciatica is the result of some irritation or damage to the sciatic nerve. This nerve originates in the lower segments of the spine. Therefore the pain, which seems to affect any or all of the area from the lower back down through the buttock, hip and thigh, can be the result of pressure at the root of the nerve. A damaged disc in the spine may be responsible. Or the spine may be pushed slightly out of normal alignment by arthritis. Or osteoporosis (a loss of calcium in the bones) of the spine may permit enough change in the bones so that pressure is exerted on the nerve.

Some toxic (poisoning) condition can be responsible. So, at times, can diabetes or gout. Infection in some remote part of the body can be responsible.

Your doctor, by making tests which you may think are far removed from your problem, may find that lurking infection, or by X-ray discover osteoporosis or arthritis of the spine, and then be able to give you some real relief.

In some instances he may have to refer you to a neurologist. If a damaged disc is involved, surgery may, occasionally, be the ultimate solution. Sciatica can be made to yield but only if you find the basic cause.

Is it dangerous to sit in a closed, parked car with the motor running?

Decidedly yes. Any leakage of exhaust gases into the car will contain carbon monoxide, which is deadly even in very low concentrations.

When the car is moving, there is enough draft to help a good bit. But even in a moving car, beware of keeping all the windows closed, unless there is some other form of ventilation.

Watch for moisture condensing on the inside of the windows. That is a sign of inadequate ventilation. If two or more people are in the car, you are using up oxygen faster than if there is only one, and hence more danger.

In bumper-to-bumper traffic, if windows are closed, do not open the ventilator on the dashboard, as it will pick up monoxide from the car ahead.

How can you guard against carbon monoxide in the home?

The first rule is to make sure that anything which burns fuel is properly vented. There must be a chimney or vent to carry fumes directly outdoors.

The greatest danger of carbon monoxide poisoning is in small hunting or vacation cabins or shacks, when oil or portable gas heaters are used without venting. In an amazingly short time, the heater has used up a good share of the available oxygen.

Combustion, in the absence of ample oxygen, results in poisonous carbon monoxide instead of the inert carbon dioxide which is not poisonous.

Ventilation is the *only* sure protection against monoxide.

Remember that carbon monoxide is invisible and has no odor. True, if you smell fumes from the furnace, you may well suspect that some monoxide might be escaping too, but you can't smell monoxide.

If in an enclosed place you begin to feel drowsy, be suspicious. Monoxide may be present. Once drowsiness comes, unconsciousness follows quickly, and then death in a matter of minutes.

Continued *slight* exposure to monoxide can cause headaches. I have in mind a chef who had persistent headaches. A clogged vent was found in the kitchen. With ventilation restored, his headaches promptly ceased.

What is the best way to treat a burn?

The quickest (and also the most effective) first aid is to keep the burned area in water. Use ordinary tap water, not ice water. It is astonishing how quickly this stops the pain.

If you take the burned hand (or whatever) out of the water too soon, the pain will commence again. Sometimes it may be necessary to wait an hour or so for a severe burn to stop paining.

Experience shows that some of the old-fashioned remedies — butter, grease, salve, etc. — are of no particular benefit, and they can be harmful, in that if the burn is severe enough to require medical or hospital treatment, the greasy or sticky stuff must then be removed.

If a burn is at all extensive, call a doctor at once. When as much as 10 per cent of the body's skin surface is burned, even if it is only a first degree burn, there is sufficient shock, as well as the body's need to throw off poisons from the burned tissues, to warrant medical attention.

With a severe and extensive burn (as with a child) if there is any waiting for medical help, getting the burned victim into a bathtub of tap-temperature water will relieve pain. Such a patient should be wrapped in a clean bed sheet when it is time to be moved — a dry sheet, not a wet one, as the dry sheet will be more effective in preventing germs from reaching the burned tissues.

Any other attempt at home treatment of a burn, except trivial ones, usually does more harm than good.

Can mumps cause sterility?

If mumps "goes down," and both testicles are affected, it can cause sterility. Once it has happened, nothing can be done to correct it. If only one testicle is involved, fertility will remain.

Please write about cystic fibrosis of the pancreas. Can anything be done for it?

Cystic fibrosis is a mean and baffling disease that has been known only for the last two or three decades. It usually affects the pancreas, but involves other parts of the body as well.

It occurs about once in every 2,000 or 3,000 people, apparently on a hereditary basis. If both parents happens to be "carriers" of the trait, the chances are about one in four that a child will have it.

Because the disease has been recognized for such a relatively short time, there are a great many things we do not know about it. How much can we do to combat it? Can we prevent it? We don't know.

It is a disorder affecting the glands which excrete fluids such as mucous, sweat and digestive enzymes. The patient has difficulty in digesting food (the products of the pancreas being necessary for digestion). Often the lungs and air passages are clogged with a sticky phlegm. Infection (flu, pneumonia or others) are hence a potential threat.

Carefully-chosen diets, antibiotics to ward off infection, and various medications to combat congestion in breathing are helpful measures.

However, there is no point in mincing words. Cystic fibrosis is dangerous. It is not contagious.

Last winter my entire family came down with flu, one after the other. Are there any precautionary measures we can take to avoid a repetition?

Yes, several, in addition to having flu vaccine in the fall.

Some, such as the first rule, will apply to virulent infection in the household: Isolate the sick one. Keep him in his room, and don't let others visit him.

Be sure there are plenty of tissues to cover the mouth while coughing, wiping the nose, etc. The used ones should be put in a paper bag, and disposed of by burning.

In the case of flu and other respiratory diseases, the germs are transmitted in droplets of moisture. You don't see anything when a patient coughs, but the tiny droplets are there. Let's go back to the old example of breathing on your glasses to moisten them enough for cleaning. That gives you an idea of how much moisture is present.

Talking, and even ordinary breathing, will scatter these germs, but not as far as a cough.

Anyone caring for a patient gains added safety by wearing a face mask, which can be improvised from an old handkerchief. It's simple, yet it makes a difference.

Don't touch the bed unless it is absolutely necessary. Besides avoiding actual contact, you automatically thus stay pretty well out of sneeze or cough range.

Wash your hands frequently, and always immediately after leaving the sick room. Viruses apparently cannot survive very long except in an environment which exactly suits them. If you have picked up the germs on your fingers, it probably does little good to wash your hands 15 or 30 minutes later.

Everyone in the household should get ample rest. Avoid fatigue. A rested person has better resistance against invading germs.

Is it possible to have basal metabolism determined by a blood test?

Rather loosely speaking, yes. Basal metabolism is determined by measuring the amount of air (oxygen) you use.

The P.B.I., or "protein-bound iodine" test, is a blood test which is very accurate. It isn't exactly a "basal metabolism test," but its purpose is essentially the same.

Other blood tests which similarly give useful data involving metabolism are the T3, which measures the uptake of radioactive iodine, and one called the thyroxine binding globulin determination.

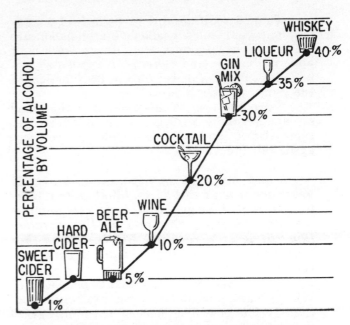

ALCOHOLIC CONTENT OF BEVERAGES

Recently a friend of mine began drinking and has continued for over two months. I doubt that he will live long enough to get cirrhosis of the liver. What alcohol content can the body tolerate at one time?

He drinks beer every day until 5 o'clock, and then drinks two fifths of liquor in highball form before midnight. Your answer may help me convey to him the danger of drinking at this rate.

He must have worked up to this enormous amount of alcohol over a period of time — perhaps unknown to you.

If you can get him to see his problem you'll be doing him a favor indeed, because he is in grave danger.

The amount of alcohol the body can tolerate varies somewhat with the individual and his size, but it is generally believed that the body can dispose of about an ounce an hour — not that it is safe or sensible to attempt that maximum.

But quite aside from the toxic effects of alcohol, most problem drinkers don't eat well or regularly, and the lack of suitable food not only increases the risk of cirrhosis but aggravates the poisonous effect of alcohol on brain, nervous system, stomach and body in general.

What are the symptoms of lead poisoning? Can it result from cleaning auto parts with gasoline?

I wonder if my 16-year-old son could have gotten it when he was repairing his car. He became quite sick, especially with headaches, lost weight and looked pale.

Lead poisoning can be caused by breathing the fumes of or handling gasoline which contains tetra-ethyl lead.

There are different degrees of lead poisoning, but your son's headaches and pallor are among the usual symptoms. Others are loss of appetite, nausea and neuritis. A typical sign is a bluish-gray discoloration at the junction of the gums and teeth.

Since the lead is absorbed into the blood stream, virtually all organs can be affected to some degree, and red blood cells can be damaged, causing anemia.

I had my first smallpox vaccination 11 years ago when I was 20, and had quite a reaction from it. I assume that I am now immune for the rest of my life, and another vaccination will never be required. But because of that experience I rather fear getting a polio vaccination.

You, along with too many people, still believe that a vaccination gives lifelong protection. It does not. The level of immunity gradually wanes, and for the more dangerous diseases, booster shots should be continued every few years — smallpox, tetanus, polio, etc. The boosters rarely cause the reactions which sometimes accompany the original inoculations, but they effectively bring protection up to full effectiveness.

For the basic inoculations which everyone should have, and the schedule for boosters, see the chart in the front of the book.

I recollect a letter from an elderly woman who insisted that she didn't need a smallpox booster because she had been vaccinated as a child, and she still had a scar. The presence of the scar means nothing. Many an oldster with a scar will have a "take" if revaccinated, which means that immunity had been lost.

In addition to the childhood inoculations, people are rightly becoming more aware of the value of influenza vaccine.

For full protection, the original flu vaccine should be given, originally, in two doses a month apart. Then a single booster once a year maintains good protection. An extra booster is advisable if a flu epidemic is known to be developing.

Flu vaccine for everyone is not yet being recommended. It is recommended — and I strongly urge it — for (1) all pregnant women; the elderly or anyone in fragile health, with particular emphasis on those with any chronic respiratory troubles; all who are in critical occupations, such as police and firemen, nurses and others in health fields (including physicians!).

The question of whether flu vaccine is advisable for children is not settled. Perhaps the best I can suggest is that circumstances in individual cases may best govern the decision.

Is it true that three days after a vaccination, the place should be wiped, or alcohol applied to it? My doctor says nothing should be put on it, but mothers of other children in my neighborhood say you should.

It's best not to cover a vaccination with anything, not even a gauze bandage, nor the plastic shields that were being used 30 or 40 years ago. Reason? The shields did no particular good and were a nuisance. And gauze can stick to the scab, break it loose, and thus delay healing.

If there happens to be considerable discharge from the vaccinated area, it is all right — in fact it's a good idea — to dab the skin *around* the scab with soap and water or with alcohol, just to keep it clean. But don't wipe across the scab itself, for fear of cracking it or pulling it loose.

It is not unsual to develop some fever after a smallpox vaccination. Children are quite likely to have more fever than an adult. They react a little harder to many things, but they get over them faster, too, as a rule.

If a severe and pussy reaction occurs, the doctor may very well choose to put a protective pad over it.

I have a frozen shoulder and would like to know what to do for it. Nothing so far has done any good, and I have had it for a long time.

A "frozen" shoulder is one that is too stiff or too painful to move, but I'm afraid that too many people have the idea that nothing can be done about such a shoulder (or other joint).

The longer such a joint remains "frozen," the more difficult it will be to get it moving again. Still, it often can be restored to some activity if you are willing to do the right things, or have the right things done to it, and will endure some pain.

What causes a "frozen" joint? Sometimes injury — such as a dislocation or fracture; sometimes bursitis; sometimes arthritis; sometimes the aftermath of having to keep the joint in one position, without moving, for a certain length of time, as with a broken collar bone. Or removal of a breast leaves the shoulder area very tender for some time. Such patients are warned to move the arm and shoulder, even though it hurts, to avoid a "frozen" shoulder.

The trouble actually is not so much in the joint itself as in tissues surrounding the joint. Adhesions (clinging together of tissues) from lack of movement can occur. There may be irritation from certain tendons riding over the joint.

How to correct it? Physical manipulation of the joint, under anesthesia, to loosen the "frozen" tissues is one way. Application of heat, plus the patient's own efforts to move the joint gradually, is another. Sometimes surgery is required to release adhesions and free trapped tendons.

The patient almost always must make up

his mind that it is going to be painful, especially in the beginning. The discomfort will lessen as the "frozen" joint recovers the ability to move normally. If you look for an "easy" or painless cure, there isn't much reason to expect good results.

Isn't appendicitis a sort of "old-fashioned" disease that really doesn't require much attention? We certainly don't hear about such frequent appendicitis operations any more.

I will grant that years ago it was even "fashionable" to have the appendix removed, but those days are long gone.

The appendix — like tonsils — appears to have a genuine purpose, although not easy to define. It seems to play a role in antibody production and hence has a role in defense against disease.

But when it becomes infected (again like tonsils) it can cause more trouble than it is worth.

It is now estimated that 75 per cent of the severe pains in the abdomen are from an irritated appendix (other common causes being kidney stones, Fallopian tube disorders, colitis, etc.)

For some reason, appendicitis today seems actually to be less prevalent than in former years. But it still happens.

The appendix dangles from the beginning of the upper bowel, in the lower right portion of the abdomen. The classical case involves pain, nausea and vomiting; if the patient tries

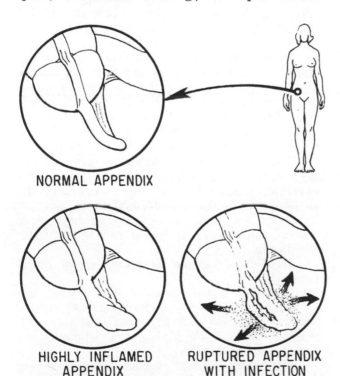

NORMAL APPENDIX

HIGHLY INFLAMED APPENDIX (APPENDICITIS REQUIRING IMMEDIATE OPERATION)

RUPTURED APPENDIX WITH INFECTION ESCAPING INTO PERITONEUM

APPENDICITIS AND RUPTURED APPENDIX

to eat, he vomits. Use of ice bag is futile; laxatives and enemas are dangerous. If in doubt, call the doctor.

Minor attacks may calm down, but in an acute attack, perforation may follow and then peritonitis. So play safe. An acute attack is still dangerous.

Where can one go to have silicone or a jelly-like substance inserted to make the breast larger? I've seen a couple of girls in show business who had this done. When I ask them where, they change the subject.

If I'd saved all the letters from women wanting some quick and easy way to enlarge the bust, I'd have a trunkful. Mainly, they inquire about three methods:

1. Is there some hormone that you can take or rub on? — I know of no effective method in this direction.

2. Will exercise help? — Only to the extent that exercises improve posture — although this can be a distinctly useful factor.

3. What about silicone injections? — There is a method, used by plastic surgeons, which involves filling a specially-shaped plastic sac with silicone, and implanting it next to the chest wall. The sac can be firmly anchored to the underlying tissues so it will remain in place; the sac itself maintains dependable shape.

Obviously, this is a painstaking process, and not inexpensive.

As to injections of silicone, without the sac and its attendant surgery, that has obviously been done, possibly more abroad than in this country.

However, despite the glowing reports of its success, there are numerous problems involved. The silicone may not remain where it was injected. Sagging and loss of shape can occur. And there remains the question of what happens as this silicone moves, and what consequences may develop years later.

Please write about dropsy. Is it hereditary and can a person who has it expect to live a normal life?

The term edema is being used more often today than dropsy, but they signify the same thing — accumulation of fluids in tissues of the body.

As you doubtless know, the body is made up in large part of water. Blood is water with a complex variety of cells and chemicals in it. Water is constantly in use by the body to collect and then discharge impurities. Water keeps food in a fluid state as it passes through the digestive tract. And so on.

When too much fluid accumulates in some part of the body, that is dropsy or edema. There are many causes — heart disease, liver or kidney disease, and others.

If the heart is weak, circulation of the blood is not as brisk as it should be. Fluid tends to settle sluggishly somewhere, often in the legs and ankles. Or impaired circulation from some cause other than a heart ailment may, of course, do the same thing.

Edema of the abdomen is quite common with cirrhosis of the liver. Certain lung conditions may cause fluid to accumulate there. And all these are merely samples. There are many more.

Thus you can see that I cannot answer your question very specifically without knowing what is causing the dropsy in your particular case. If the cause can be corrected, then the condition of edema can be brought to an end. In other instances, it may be necessary to accept dropsy as a chronic condition, and your goal is to keep it under control.

One example is the patient with heart trouble who is put on low-salt diet. Salt (the sodium in it) has an affinity for water, tending to hold it. You know how soggy salt can get in humid weather! If we can keep the amount of salt in the body at a low level, then less fluid is retained in the body.

Diuretics, or drugs to release water from the body, also are used. But as you can see, each case must be judged by itself.

Dropsy is not hereditary.

What about the after effects of cobalt treatments? Through such treatments and surgery, my sister has been cured of cancer of the uterus.

However, for a number of months now she has had diarrhea badly, and is sick and tired most of the time.

When heavy radiation treatment is required — and it saves many lives, of course — the patient should not expect it to be a simple or casual process.

The purpose is to direct an intense beam of rays at the cancer (whether from a cobalt unit, or a high-voltage X-ray tube is immaterial, since the rays are the same.)

Since the cancerous cells are "sick" or defective, they are destroyed more readily than normal cells.

However, the rays are so powerful that they damage healthy cells, too, although not to such a degree. That is the delicate part of the use of X-ray: To deliver enough to destroy the cancer, but not enough to do irreparable harm to other cells. That is why heavy shields are used, and the rays are focused very sharply, so they will strike only where they are needed.

If the bladder and bowel are irradiated, one of the side effects is just the sort you describe. A low-residue diet (to reduce irritation of the bowel) and appropriate medications to control cramps and diarrhea are necessary until the cells are restored to normal.

While the body is involved in the process of returning to normal, it is under continued strain, and the patient may feel "sick and tired" some of the time.

My doctor wanted me to take a cortisone drug but I refused. I am concerned about its side effects because I want to have another baby in the near future, and for other obvious reasons. Could you recommend some other drug?

I think you are confusing what MAY happen when cortisone is used for long periods with what will or won't happen from moderate use.

You can be sure that your doctor is perfectly aware of what side effects to guard against. I cannot see that moderate use of it has anything to do with another baby, and I don't know any other obvious reasons. Cortisone, with proper medical supervision, is a beneficial medication.

I would like to know about D.T.'s. Can anything be done unless the person is willing? Is it dangerous?

D.T.'s, or delirium tremens is the end point of too much indulgence in strong drink. It involves jitters, nervousness, hallucinations, staggering gait — you name it. It's there.

Whether the victim is dangerous to others depends on circumstances and on what hallucinations he may have. It is certainly dangerous (and desperately uncomfortable) for the victim himself, since there is bound to be physical damage from the amount of drinking needed to bring on delirium tremens. Cirrhosis of the liver is the one that comes first to mind.

Please write about anesthesia. Some of my friends and I fear it so much we refuse to have necessary surgery. I do not worry about anything I understand, but the patient rarely sees the anesthetist. I had surgery recently, and was not prepared for the anesthetic and its effect. Here are my specific questions. . . .

Why is an enema given as part of the preparation even when, as in my case, the operation is not internal? Mine was orthopedic surgery on the lower extremities.

It's a good idea to clean out the colon, since loss of control of the bowel can occur under anesthesia.

Why is a "saline solution" given intravenously?

The salt water, injected into a vein, bolsters the blood pressure which tends to decline under anesthesia. An injection also is a convenient method of giving nourishment and various medications.

Pentothal brings unconsciousness very fast. Is it a hypnotic drug? Does the patient just sleep or does he respond to commands? Is he apt to be talkative?

Pentothal brings unconsciousness rapidly.

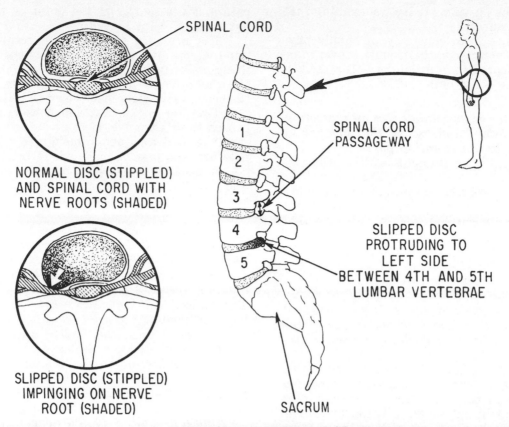

'SLIPPED' INTERVERTEBRAL DISC

Left: Cross-section of vertebra and disc, viewed from above. Right: The lower spine, with nerve roots omitted.

Depending on the amount given, the patient might be talkative (it is one of the drugs which is used in small quantities as a "truth serum"). Although it doesn't necessarily force the truth, it makes lying difficult. With increased quantity the patient responds to commands; a little more, and he "goes to sleep" entirely, in which case he won't respond.

What is the purpose of the tube in the throat? Should it be inserted while the patient is awake, even though some discomfort is involved?

It has two main purposes. One is to prevent the tongue from blocking the airway in the back of the throat. The other is to permit "intratracheal anesthesia," which is used in some instances. There are times when the tube should be inserted before anesthesia; other times the reverse.

Following surgery, what causes extreme and prolonged rhythmic spasms, or the "dry heaves," as it is called?

Relaxation of the colon may permit gaseous distension, and the "dry heaves" are Nature's way of trying to get rid of the gas. The condition is more likely to occur after surgery on the intestinal tract. Giving oxygen at termination of anesthesia tends to lessen the heaves.

I would like information about a slipped disc.

Several weeks ago I picked up a heavy object and had the feeling that something pulled loose in my back. I put a plaster on my back but it just doesn't seem to get well.

Now every time I try to pick up something I have severe pain in my back and down my leg.

Should I go to my family physician or to a specialist?

The "slipped disc" probably has had more publicity than is good for us, because it makes people lose sight of the fact that many other things can go wrong with the back.

Discs are pads of cartilage which lie between the bones of the spine. "Damaged disc" is a better term because a disc is unlikely to be forced out of normal position unless it first is damaged or ruptured.

You may, it is true, have damaged a disc. It is even more likely, however, that you strained or even tore a ligament or muscle in your back which causes pain when you lift.

The result of this can be to put pressure on a nerve at the point at which it branches out from the spinal column, and that in turn can explain the pain which radiates down your leg.

Taping or use of a brace often can prevent the pain, along with giving the damaged tissues time to heal without being strained again.

The back has a large network of muscles and it takes considerable familiarity with the muscle pattern to put the taping or brace in just the right position. It isn't something that you can do yourself.

My advice is to consult your family physician. If, in your case, the trouble proves to be more complicated than usual, he will refer you to a specialist — an orthopedist.

Please give some reliable tips on protection from trichinosis. I understand that one has to be very careful about eating pork.

One must be careful not to eat *insufficiently cooked* pork.

Trichinosis is caused by an almost invisibly small worm (the trichina worm), a parasite.

When a worm hatches in the intestinal tract, it produces a new generation of tiny worms which then work their way through the body and finally, after much irritation, become "encysted," or nest down in muscle fibers.

They may remain thus snoozing for a long time, but if the meat in which they have nested is ultimately eaten again, they emerge in the digestive tract and the whole process is repeated.

Pork is the principal meat involved in this disease because, primarily, garbage is often fed to pigs, and garbage can contain infected meat — and pigs will eat meat. (Cattle, of course, don't eat meat, hence do not pick up the trichina infection.)

There is one sure way of avoiding trichinosis: Insist that pork (or meat from any animal which will eat meat) be thoroughly cooked. That will kill the worms and keep you safe from trichinosis. That means that pork should be cooked until it is gray all the way through, not pink.

Informed estimates are that from 15 to 20 per cent of Americans encounter trichinosis at one time or another. Sometimes it may be mild and symptoms are not recognized, but in some instances it can be serious.

I sleep with my arms above my head. Is this harmful?

No, but by pinching certain nerves or large blood vessels it may cause tingling or numbness in your fingers. Sleep whichever way is most comfortable.

Please write about calcium spurs. After an extensive examination, including X-rays, brain wave test, etc., a neurologist diagnosed my severe head and scalp pains as originating from "discs in the neck that have spurs on them." He advised traction.

The "spurs" in this case are overgrowths of the neck bones — that is, of the edges of some of these bones. This is a quite common occurrence as we grow older.

Should these overgrowths be in such position as to put pressure on certain of the nerves radiating from the spine, the result can be pain, not necessarily at the point of pressure, but at some point served by the nerve.

The pressure on the nerve results in an impulse reaching the brain that is the same as though the painful situation were occurring elsewhere. These pains need not seem to be in the head; they fairly often seem to be the arms.

Traction is the first and conservative approach to this trouble. If the bones of the neck can thus be drawn apart enough to relieve the pressure, the pain is lessened. If traction does not succeed, then surgery may be necessary. The goal is to take the pressure off those nerves and to relax tense muscles in the neck.

I have trouble with stiffness in my arm. A doctor X-rayed my elbow and it showed joint mice. Would surgery correct this?

Joint mice are tiny bits of calcium in the area, the result of infection or other irritation. The "mice," in fact, represent Nature's attempt at healing.

In themselves, the "mice" are not ordinarily painful, and the discomfort and stiffness may be due instead to the original irritation. If necessary the "mice" can, however, be flushed out or picked out surgically.

I am a woman of 40 and desperately seeking help. I am an alcoholic. Don't tell me to go to AA because that would mean exposing myself to my family. I would rather die.

I have tried many times on my own, but to no avail. I have heard there is a potent drug that can help if the patient is willing and really wants to stop. Is this true?

"AA" means Alcoholics Anonymous, and the "Anonymous" means just what it says, so I do not see why going to AA would expose your problem to your family.

I have discussed this with AA members, and one of the penetrating replies was, "And just how is she going to explain it to her family, anyway, when she is sober all the time?"

You see, secret alcoholics characteristically think they have everybody fooled. Drinkers who have been through the mill tell me this is very seldom true. Almost always it is a case of friends and family pretending they don't know, when they do.

AA achieves its finest results with people who voluntarily and sincerely seek its help, and I think you genuinely want help. Why not try it?

Yes, there are potent drugs which make a person violently ill if alcohol is consumed. This sounds foolproof but it isn't. The flaw is that if a person really wants another drink, he always can find one way or another to stop taking the drug. The real cure lies deeper: Helping the patient develop a compelling desire to quit.

The drug, however, is useful in some cases, but it needs close supervision by a physician.

What causes pyorrhea? Is there a cure? My 37-year-old son has this trouble. He has consulted a number of dentists but they don't all agree. Some want to extract only a few teeth and leave the others for an abutment. Personally I feel all the teeth should be removed if they are diseased.

I can't agree that all his teeth should be removed. Perhaps so, perhaps not. It depends on the condition of those teeth.

I've consulted Dr. Alfred E. Seyler, a dentist of considerable prominence:

I'll give you the information he gave me. But first, what is pyorrhea? A disease of the gums, rather than of the teeth. It is quite possible (although perhaps not probable) that someone without any cavities may still have pyorrhea.

Germs congregate, not in the gums at first, but in the crevices between or on the surface of the teeth. As this continues, the gums become inflamed, at the tooth margins. There may be little or no pain. But as the germ colonies increase, they work down below the surface, along the tooth, and the gum recedes.

There is no single germ. There are many varieties. There is no drug that can "cure pyorrhea." There's no easy way of stopping it.

Yet it is not a hopeless problem, either. We have antibiotics, and we also have modern techniques.

Having the teeth cleaned by a dentist every so often is certainly the best method of preventing pyorrhea, because it removes the tartar or calculus which is such a breeding ground for germs.

What causes migraine headaches and can they be prevented? I was 13 when I had my first one.

When I get one I first start seeing black spots, then white jagged lines appear for about 30 minutes. Then I can see again but I get terrible headaches and the light hurts my eyes.

The cause is not absolutely established, but it is known to involve an overdilation of the blood vessels in the brain. Tense people, perfectionists who have to have everything just so, are the more usual victims of migraines, and they tend to begin from the very early teens to the mid-20's. By the age of 50, most people have passed the "migraine age," but that's a long time to wait.

Stopping a migraine isn't often successful, but various drugs and their combinations, largely based on ergotamine tartrate, can ward off or ease an attack — if taken in time.

This means that the patient must learn to recognize the signs that precede an attack. These vary from person to person. Being irritable, or forgetful, or depressed or the like are signs for some. Others notice that their fingers swell a little. They may get ringing noises in the ears. Becoming too tired, or upset and angry, or a feeling of being under pressure are things that help trigger an attack.

The spots and flashes of light are quite common with migraine. Some people have temporary "blind spots" for a short time.

Please write about tic douloureux and the possible effectiveness of Vitamin B$_{12}$ injections.

Tic douloureux is, in its severe form, one of the most agonizing pains known to man. It is a neuralgia which affects the nerves of the face and head, which is a sensitive area. Its cause is not known. Its behavior is not altogether predictable.

It is a periodic pain, often subsiding or becoming less intense at night.

Simple movements or contacts can set off new attacks — the facial movement when you chew, touching the face as in washing, etc.

Personality factors seem to be very important and such questions as the patient's feelings of dependency, his environment and psychological state should be investigated. Altering his attitude can be very helpful.

The B complex vitamins seem to have a tonic effect on nerve tissue and this can be helpful, but it is doubtful that B$_{12}$, being only a fraction of the complex, would have any more effect than B$_1$ (or thiamine) or the whole complex.

In milder cases, simple pain medication can provide relief. Brief inhalation of trichlorethylene (breathing from a small amount poured on a cloth or a handkerchief) gives emergency relief.

I am sterile. A friend told me that it is now possible to treat such people. My wife wants very much to have children. My doctor says I cannot.

Sterility, like so many other conditions, doesn't always result from the same cause. Therefore, while sometimes it can be corrected, often it can't. For example mumps, if affecting both testes, may (not always will) cause complete sterility and nothing can be done about it.

The presence of viable (living) sperm is the fundamental factor. Sometimes the cells are not viable. Sometimes they are inactive — lack the power to move around. Or there may be very few cells.

In other cases, the sperm may be viable yet because of some physiological defect cannot get out. In such cases, surgical correction may be possible.

Examination of sperm samples can give a good clue as to whether anything can be done, or whether, for example, hormone treatment can help.

Since you have been examined, and your doctor has given such a gloomy report, my advice would be to think about adoption.

Index

Bold Face Numbers Indicate Illustrations

IMPORTANT VITAMIN SOURCES

Carotene (which converts to Vitamin A—Milk, butter, egg yolk, yellow vegetables, fish oils.

Vitamin B1 (thiamin)—Green vegetables, whole cereals, pork, liver.

Vitamin B2 (riboflavin)—Milk, meat.

Niacin (nicotinic acid)—Milk and meat.

Vitamin B6—Meat, grain, vegetables.

Folic acid—Green vegetables.

Vitamin B12—Meat, and especially liver.

Vitamin C (ascorbic acid)—Citrus fruits and juices, tomato juice, raw tomatoes are the primary sources, which explains the emphasis on breakfast juices every day. Cooking destroys Vitamin C, but canned or frozen juices are excellent.

Vitamin D—This is called the "sunshine vitamin" because ultraviolet light (sunshine) is necessary to create it from fish oils, butter, egg yolk. It is particularly vital for good bone formation and prevention of rickets. That is why fishliver oil is given to babies, and why it is important to children who get little sunshine.

Vitamin E (tocopherol)—In wheat germ oil and other vegetable oils. Despite claims made for Vitamin E, there is little scientific evidence that people develop deficiency.

Vitamin K and Vitamin P, while useful at times as medications for special purposes, require no dietary precautions.

CALORIE CONTENT OF DIET-WRECKING SNACK FOODS

FOOD	AMOUNT	CALORIES
Chocolate bar	1 small bar	155
Chocolate creams	1 average size	50
Cookies	1 medium size	75
Doughnut	1 plain	135
Banana	1 large	100
Peach	1 medium size	50
Apple	1 medium size	75
Raisins	½ cup	200
Popcorn	1 cup popped	55
Potato chips	8–10 or ½ cup	100
Peanuts or pistachio nuts	1	5
Walnuts, pecans, filberts, or cashews	4 whole or 1 tbsp. chopped	40
Brazil nuts	1	50
Butternuts	1	25
Peanut butter	1 tbsp.	100

FOOD	AMOUNT	CALORIES
Olives	1	10
Pickles	1 large sour	10
	1 average sweet	15
Ice cream	½ cup	200
Chocolate-nut sundae		270
Ice cream soda		225
Chocolate malted milk	1 glass	450
Eggnog (without liquor)	1 glass	235
Carbonated beverages	6 oz. or 1 bottle	80

ALCOHOLIC BEVERAGES		CALORIES
Beer	8 oz. glass	120
Wine	1 wine glass	75
Gin	1 jigger	115
Rum	1 jigger	125
Whiskey	1 jigger	120
Brandy	1 brandy glass	80
Cocktail	1 cocktail glass	150

GASTROINTESTINAL (DIGESTIVE) TRACT

Food works its way through stomach and intestines, is worked on by juices manufactured in various organs (like the liver and pancreas), then absorbed mainly thru intestinals walls; residue is excreted through the rectum.

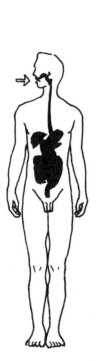

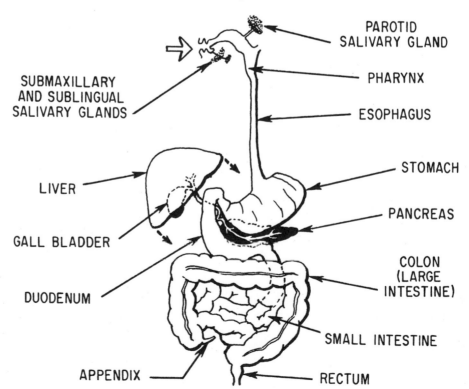

PAROTID SALIVARY GLAND

SUBMAXILLARY AND SUBLINGUAL SALIVARY GLANDS

PHARYNX

ESOPHAGUS

LIVER

STOMACH

PANCREAS

GALL BLADDER

COLON (LARGE INTESTINE)

DUODENUM

SMALL INTESTINE

APPENDIX

RECTUM